362.198
GLE

When Your
Loved One
Has Dementia

When Your
Loved One
Has Dementia

A Simple Guide for Caregivers

Joy A. Glenner, Jean M. Stehman,
Judith Davagnino, Margaret J. Galante,
and Martha L. Green

*The George G. Glenner Alzheimer's Family Centers, Inc.
San Diego, California*

The Johns Hopkins University Press
Baltimore and London

© 2005 The Johns Hopkins University Press
All rights reserved. Published 2005
Printed in the United States of America on acid-free paper
9 8 7 6 5 4 3 2 1

The Johns Hopkins University Press
2715 North Charles Street
Baltimore, Maryland 21218-4363
www.press.jhu.edu

Library of Congress Cataloging-in-Publication Data

When your loved one has dementia : a simple guide for caregivers / Joy A.
Glenner . . . [et al.].
     p.   cm.
   Includes index.
   ISBN 0-8018-8113-7 (hardcover : alk. paper) — ISBN 0-8018-8114-5
(pbk. : alk. paper)
   1. Senile dementia—Patients—Home care.   2. Senile dementia—
Patients—Family relationships.   3. Caregivers.   I. Glenner, Joy A., 1930–
   RC523.W466 2005
   362.198′976831—dc22

                                                            2004024466

A catalog record for this book is available from the British Library.

Contents

Introduction

The six chapters of *When Your Loved One Has Dementia* emphasize the importance of good communication with your family member as a method of ensuring a better quality of life for both you and your partner. A glossary is included to assist you in understanding unfamiliar words. The handbook is written in a conversational style that, we hope, will reassure and support you as you grow in your caregiving role. You can grow in this process if you try to look at it as a partnership with your ill family member and with others—friends, family members, and care professionals—who will help you in supporting roles.

When Your Loved One Has Dementia emphasizes ongoing communication with your ill family member. We often refer to your family member as your "partner." Throughout the course of a progressive dementing illness, regular and natural two-way verbal and nonverbal communication will help you determine care needs and may help you remain close to each other—as true partners. Remaining close to your partner and maintaining ties with family and friends can be an effective support system. If you are not close or have grown apart over the years, time as a caregiver for your partner can be a good opportunity to "mend fences."

In this book we also use the term **patient.** As the disease progresses, initiation of communication, needs *assessment,* and the implementation of care will become more and more your responsibility. Your partner will communicate with you through actions more than words, yet you will still need to be able to understand what he or she may be trying to convey. Knowing your partner well will help with ongoing assessment as the disease becomes more severe and conversation becomes more and more nonverbal. Words that may be unfamiliar are in italics and are found in the glossary.

The better you understand the needs and feelings your family member expresses verbally and nonverbally, the easier the caregiving process will be and the more confident you will feel about your role as caregiver.

When Your
Loved One
Has Dementia

1 Understanding and Acceptance

Goal: This chapter will help you identify the symptoms of a dementing illness. It will also help you understand the *pathology* of *Alzheimer disease* (AD) and the latest research on it. It will suggest ways in which you and your partner can become or remain close while adjusting to the changes that lie ahead.

Early Warning Signs

We all forget things once in a while, more often as we get older. Mild forgetfulness is normal. But where does "normal" end and a problem begin? It is often very difficult to tell.

Benign forgetfulness is just what it implies: it is benign, or not harmful, and it is a normal part of aging.

Mild cognitive impairment (MCI) means there is some decline in memory, but the person can still cope fairly well in everyday life. It is not normal aging. Many of those diagnosed with MCI decline and develop Alzheimer disease, but many do not become noticeably worse.

Dementia is a general term meaning a global loss of intellectual functioning and normal alertness caused by *disease* or injury to the brain. AD is the most common cause of dementia.

Box 1-1 lists some examples of early warning signs.

Box 1-1. Early Warning Signs

The descriptions of Mr. Carpenter's problems are examples of benign forgetfulness, mild cognitive impairment, and mild dementia.

Benign forgetfulness
- Mr. Carpenter is eighty years old and in good health. He has begun to be concerned, however, that he is becoming forgetful.
- He keeps notes to himself folded in his wallet. On them he writes phone numbers he uses frequently and things he wishes to do that day. He refers to the notes frequently so he will remember tasks when he reads them. He then crosses off each one as he completes it.
- He frequently repeats stories he has already told but usually catches himself and apologizes.
- Mr. Carpenter does not have an abnormal memory problem. He makes adaptations to help him remember when he temporarily forgets. He still functions very well without help.

Mild cognitive impairment (MCI)
- Mr. Carpenter gradually forgets to read the notes in his wallet, though he continues to plan and to write them. He repeats stories without realizing he is repeating.
- He then makes a medical appointment for a cognitive assessment because of his new concerns.
- After the evaluation of his problems confirms MCI, Mr. Carpenter decides to move to a retirement community that provides meals and van service. His losses are now noticeable, but he is still able to assess them, and he adapts well by making appropriate lifestyle changes.

Mild dementia
- Mr. Carpenter has trouble driving. He gets lost frequently and avoids freeways because he cannot drive well enough anymore. When he almost hits someone with his car, he stops driving.

- He starts forgetting ingredients when he cooks, and he burns things on the stove.
- Mr. Carpenter may have dementia if his symptoms progress. If he becomes unable to plan ahead, regularly forgets to do routine daily activities, and forgets recent events and is unable to recall them if reminded, he may have a problem. He will probably be unable to live independently. He may decide to move to an assisted living community.

Understanding the Symptoms You May See

Try to assess your partner's symptoms objectively. This can be difficult. It is natural to want to deny or fight these changes, to "protect" someone you love. But denial or trying to correct behaviors improperly can damage your relationship and make life more stressful for both of you.

Your objective assessment will help you and your physician obtain an accurate *diagnosis* and will guide you in daily life with your partner. To make an objective assessment, you must first understand and be able to identify the basic symptoms of a dementing illness. They are the symptoms observable in everyone who has a dementing illness.

The basic symptoms of dementia result from damage to all of the mental functions that we use in daily life. Remember, dementia is global brain damage. The symptoms are, of course, mild at first, but they become very severe if the dementia is progressive (such as with AD). They are not behavior problems. The brain damage causes these basic symptoms, and they result in difficult behavior.

We developed a memory cue to help you remember the basic symptoms: "Mr. [or Mrs.] Palmer has dementia." Each letter of the word *PALMER* stands for a symptom. The letter *P* helps you remember two symptoms, and so does the *R*; the rest of the letters stand for a single symptom (box 1-2).

Box 1-2. The Basic Symptoms of Dementia:
The PALMER Memory Cue

Perception and organization of movement
Attention span
Language ability
Memory
Emotional control
Reasoning and judgment

The basic symptoms of dementia include problems with:

1. Perception and organization of movement

Perception is understanding or interpreting the environment. It is our understanding of what we see, hear, feel, taste, or smell. For example, a person may be able to see things very clearly and hear even very faint sounds but be unable to recognize or correctly interpret what he or she is seeing or hearing.

Agnosia is the loss of visual perception, the inability to recognize familiar objects and surroundings.

Mrs. Jameson rearranged the furniture. Mr. Jameson then had trouble finding his favorite chair because it was not where it used to be. When Mrs. Jameson pointed it out, guided him to it, and had him touch it, he recognized it. He had trouble with visual perception.

Organization of movement is the ability to move ourselves and other objects about.

Mr. Jameson also had trouble sitting in the chair. He would sometimes kneel on the chair instead of sitting or would not sit all the way down—he would lower himself part way and then get back up. When

Mrs. Jameson gave him step-by-step verbal cues, guided him with her hands, and reassured him that he would not fall, he sat down. He had trouble organizing his movements correctly.

2. Attention span

Attention span is the amount of time we can concentrate on a task or on what is going on around us.

Samuel loved to chop vegetables for a dinner salad each night. He would start to chop the vegetables but then would stop and walk away before they were done. His wife, Eve, decided to stay with him as he worked. Whenever he started to drift away, she reminded him that he needed to finish chopping. He then continued. She usually had to remind him two or three times. He had a very short attention span.

3. Language ability

Language ability is receptive and expressive. Receptive language ability is the ability to understand the meaning of oral (spoken) and written information. Expressive language ability is the ability to convey oral or written information to others. Loss of language ability is *aphasia*.

Susan was looking at a photo album and motioned to her sister, April (her *caregiver*), to come closer and see a photo. She tried to tell April why the picture was special but became upset because she had trouble expressing what she wanted to say. She had poor expressive language ability.

April then asked Susan questions about the picture. Susan could not understand the questions and became even more upset. She also had poor receptive language ability. April then just stated that it was a beautiful picture and that she liked it too. Susan understood this simple statement, and it did not require an answer. She calmed down.

4. Memory

Memory has three components: awareness, retention, and retrieval. We cannot remember anything if we are not aware of it first. We then have to retain it—or "keep it" in our brain in order to retrieve or recall it later—the process of "thinking." Accurate memory depends on other brain functions. For example, memory will be poor if perception and attention span are compromised.

Antonio loved to make cutting boards and other simple wood projects. He spent hours sanding and oiling or waxing projects, and he enjoyed talking to his daughter Anna about them as he worked. When she admired a finished project, however, Antonio would often say, "Who did that?" When told that he made it, he did not remember doing so but was always pleased when Anna told him he had done it. Even though he was aware of a project as he did it, he immediately forgot it. He was unable to retain and retrieve the information later. His memory was very impaired.

5. Emotional control

Emotional control is the ability to feel and stay relaxed, pleasant, and calm in normal daily life. We usually keep anger, anxiety, sadness, and other strong emotions at an acceptable level (not always, of course!) and display them only when we really need to. People with dementia have trouble doing this.

Mr. Culbertson asked the family physician to prescribe a medication to control his wife Sarah's anxiety. He was exhausted, because she became extremely anxious if he was ever out of her sight. She also was very anxious when they went out, even to the grocery store they had shopped at together for years. She became angry and frequently struck out at him if noises were too loud (such as the television or vacuum cleaner). Sarah was unable to control emotions adequately, specifically anxiety and anger.

6. Reasoning and judgment

Reasoning is putting thoughts together to form more complex thoughts and ideas. Judgment is the process of evaluating or comparing different thoughts and ideas to reach a conclusion. People with dementia have impaired reasoning and judgment.

Martin has lived in the same home for fifty years and walks around the neighborhood every day. Recently he began losing his way. The local police knew him and frequently brought him home. His son Joseph lived with him and reminded him often that he might get lost and should not walk alone. Martin always became angry and told his son that he was disrespectful, even when Joseph reminded him of the specific times he had gotten lost and the police had brought him home. Martin also accused Joseph of trying to make him a prisoner. This shocked and hurt his son, but he realized that Martin did not understand due to poor reasoning and poor judgment—the inability to reach a logical conclusion. He enrolled Martin in adult day care, where he walked with others every day. Joseph no longer left his father at home alone. He also walked with him every evening.

The Stages of Dementia

The basic PALMER symptoms will not all grow worse at the same rate. Nevertheless, clinicians and researchers recognize at least three stages of dementia (box 1-3). Use the stages as a general guide only. For example, your partner may still have good language skills (stage 1) but may have severe memory loss and loss of emotional control (late stage 2 or even stage 3).

Dorothy is generally a moderately impaired person with Alzheimer disease. Her basic symptoms have declined at different rates, however, and her husband, Larry, tries to keep her active in things she can still

Box 1-3. The Three Stages of Irreversible and Progressive Dementia

Stage 1. Onset, mild dementia
> Often this stage is deceptive, with:
>> recent memory loss and mild loss of language ability (aphasia)
>> confusion, decreased attention span
>> impaired reasoning and judgment
>> anxiety, depression, and withdrawal common
>> noticeable difficulty with Instrumental Activities of
>> Daily Living (IADLs)

Stage 2. Middle, moderate dementia
> All symptoms of stage 1 are increased, with:
>> restlessness and agitation common
>> repetitive behaviors or perseveration
>> disorientation in familiar places
>> unsteady, stiff gait (hypertonia)
>> difficulty with perception and organization of movement
>> difficulty with toileting, continence care, other Activities
>> of Daily Living (ADLs)
>> some long-term memory loss

Stage 3. Terminal, severe dementia
> Needs constant supervision and assistance, with:
>> delusions and hallucinations common
>> incontinence: first urinary, then fecal (incontinence of bowels)
>> difficulty swallowing, causing choking and aspiration
>> emaciation
>> loss of response and general awareness

do. He simplifies or takes over tasks that she can no longer do or which frustrate her.

She is very social and loves to be with others. She speaks and understands others well and can carry on great simple conversations. Her language disability is very mild. She avoids personal conversations, however, because she really cannot remember who her friends are or where she has met them before. Larry stays close by at parties to make sure she is not embarrassed. She has moderate to severe short-term memory loss.

Her long-term memory, on the other hand, is still quite good. She was a third-grade teacher for many years, and she remembers many things about her past career. The problem is that she assumes that all of the people with whom she socializes used to be in her third-grade classroom. Her reasoning ability is moderately impaired.

Dorothy attended an Alzheimer Adult Day Care Center and became attached to a friendly male patient there named Jim. She often insisted he was her husband (a delusion), even though Larry is six feet tall and Jim was far shorter and looked nothing like him. Staff members tried to reason with her, telling her that Jim's wife would be upset if she saw them spending so much time together. This made Dorothy very upset, and she was very hard to calm down. She had moderate to severe lack of judgment and had moderate to severely impaired emotional control. Larry and Jim's wife now work together to ensure that their spouses do not attend the center on the same days.

Dorothy still dresses herself with suggestions and a watchful eye from Larry. She helps prepare meals and cleans house. She loves day care, as she does every social situation. She dances beautifully to music with a staff member or fellow participant as a partner. She loves arts and crafts and cooking projects and does them beautifully. Her attention span, perception, and organization of movement are all only mildly impaired.

The Specifics of Alzheimer Disease and Other Dementing Illnesses

The History of Alzheimer Disease

Alzheimer disease is a neurological disorder or disease most common in older adults. It destroys vital brain cells, causing a global decline in the ability to function.

In 1907 a German psychiatrist, Dr. Alois Alzheimer, discovered abnormal "plaques and tangles" in the cerebral cortex, or "gray matter," the outer layer of the brain. It was called "presenile dementia" because the brain damage was first seen in patients under age sixty-five.

In 1968 three British pathologists determined that AD was not a rare disease of younger patients, but was most often, in fact, what was then termed *senility*.

The Pathology of Alzheimer Disease

There seem to be several different genes causing AD. Sometimes AD is familial (runs in families); other times it occurs randomly but more commonly with age.

In 1984 Dr. George Glenner identified a body protein associated with a gene on chromosome 21, called *beta-amyloid* protein. It is found in the brains of all patients with AD. The beta-amyloid and another protein called "tau" are responsible for causing the brain damage. Tau protein is found in the tangles (see fig. 1-1).

Statistics

- AD is the most common cause of dementia, accounting for 65 percent of those with a dementing illness.
- More than four million adults have AD.
- One out of five people over age sixty-five is affected. The rate

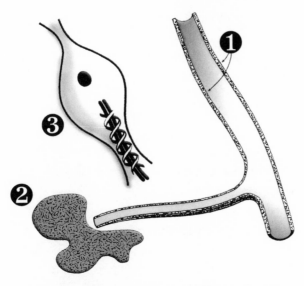

Fig. 1-1. The brain damage of Alzheimer disease. The beta-amyloid protein is taken up by the cells of blood vessels in the brain (1). A small portion of this protein breaks through blood vessels and is the primary component of abnormal plaques exterior to brain cells (2). The tau protein is the primary component of amyloid fibers in brain cells (3).

increases to nearly half of those age eighty-five and older. The disease is costing more than $100 billion a year in the United States.

- AD is the cause of more than 50 percent of nursing home admissions.

Other Dementing Illnesses

There are other dementias too, and a good diagnosis can determine if a patient has one of them. A person can have more than one type of dementia. Some types of dementia are treatable, so a good diagnosis is essential.

Other illnesses that cause dementia are numerous but are rarer than AD. More than 50 percent of persons with dementia have

AD. Patients with other dementing illnesses have similar symptoms. Also, a person may have more than one type of dementia at a time, making the *differential diagnosis* more complex. The suggestions and techniques in this book can be used with anyone with dementia.

Other progressive and untreatable dementing illnesses include:

- vascular dementia
- frontotemporal lobe dementia and Pick disease
- Creutzfeldt-Jakob disease
- Lewy body dementia
- dementia associated with Parkinson disease

The primary symptom or a common symptom of all dementias is cognitive decline. Other symptoms may also be present. A differential diagnosis will determine whether the disease is AD or another cause of dementia.

There are also treatable, or nonprogressive, dementias. It is very important to obtain an accurate diagnosis so that your partner can receive appropriate treatment. Treatable conditions include:

- Drug side effects or interactions: This is very common, so look at multiple drug use or improper dosage of prescription drugs as a first cause of the dementia. Be sure to bring all medications (including nonprescription and herbal remedies) to your partner's diagnostic evaluation.
- Poor nutrition: Frail older adults without someone to monitor their condition and provide care may have symptoms of dementia caused by poor nutrition.
- Depression: Sometimes a person will deny feeling "down" or "sad" but may experience symptoms of depression such as apathy, sleeping long hours, or having trouble sleeping. The person may express anxiety or withdraw. There is no actual brain

tissue damage, so it is referred to as a "pseudo-" (false) dementia. There may, however, be a chemical imbalance. Depression is also common with any diagnosis of dementia or another debilitating disease and can easily be treated with medication.

- Alcoholism (a severe form is Korsakoff syndrome): Alcoholism is often combined with depression and can lead to serious health problems, even death. It can be more serious with poor nutrition, if the person is weak due to illness or is taking certain types of prescription medications. If the person stops drinking alcohol, the dementia will at least not get worse and may improve.

- Hypothyroidism: The person may have unexplained weight gain, puffy face or eye areas, slowed speech, or increased sensitivity to cold. It is easily treated with medication.

- Vitamin B_{12} deficiency: Pernicious anemia is a result of the body's inability to absorb vitamin B_{12} in the diet. The person may become weak and pale and may lose weight. Injections of B_{12} will help very quickly (but not taking vitamin B_{12} by mouth).

Remember, if you see signs of dementia in daily life with your partner, be sure to tell your physician because the condition may be treatable.

Seeing the Difference: A CAT Scan

Figure 1-2 shows the difference between normal aging, AD, and vascular dementia. Cerebral atrophy (loss of cell fluids causing death of the cell) in the brain's gray matter characterizes AD. Cell atrophy occurs first in the *hippocampus*. *Ventricles* also become enlarged due to the loss of the gray matter. In vascular dementia damage is more random and occurs in other areas of the brain besides the cerebral cortex.

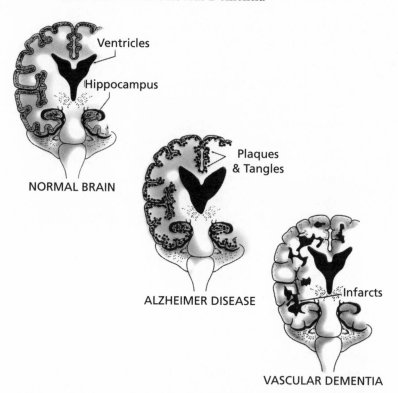

Fig. 1-2. CAT scans showing the difference between a normal brain, a brain with Alzheimer disease, and a brain with vascular dementia.

Diagnosis, Treatment, and Prevention of Alzheimer Disease

More and more progress is being made in diagnosing, treating, and even possibly preventing AD.

Diagnosis

Admitting to a problem is difficult, so getting a comprehensive evaluation and diagnosis for your partner is a big step. If you use a reputable clinic that does a thorough differential diagnosis, you can rely on that opinion. Sometimes the diagnosis will be "probable Alzheimer disease" or "progressive dementia." This is okay if you know the diagnosis was thorough and eliminated the possibility of treatable symptoms.

Good clinics can be found nationwide. The Alzheimer's Association has a referral list of chapters across the United States, or check with the National Institute on Aging, Alzheimer's Disease Education and Referral (ADEAR) (see Resources page).

Getting a differential diagnosis is the best way to determine that a person has AD. It differentiates the symptoms from other diseases, so the process is complicated, and it takes more than one visit to a clinic. The differential diagnostic process is so dependable today that the accuracy rate as measured against evidence from an *autopsy* is 90 percent. Nevertheless, AD can only be positively diagnosed at autopsy.

It is very important to get an accurate diagnosis. There *are* treatable dementing illnesses. Once you make the commitment to get a diagnosis, be sure to follow through. It is time-consuming but worth it.

Treatment and Prevention

Medications in tablet form which can temporarily slow the dementing process are now frequently prescribed, but even with these medications the disease will eventually get worse. Alzheimer disease is always progressive and lethal (fatal)—it *always* results in death.

The best treatment to date is the use of cholinesterase inhibitors. These are medications that keep the enzyme acetylcholinesterase from breaking down an important chemical, *acetylcholine,* needed to make connections between brain cells.

- Aricept (donepezil) is a commonly used cholinesterase inhibitor. Physicians are now prescribing it not just for early-stage AD but also for mild cognitive impairment.
- Other cholinesterase inhibitors are Excelon (rivastigmine) and Reminyl (galantamine). Namenda (memantine) has been approved for the treatment of moderate to severe AD. It is believed to work by regulating glutamate, an important brain chemical that may lead to brain cell death when it is produced in excessive amounts.

The inhibitors slow the progress of AD symptoms, but even with them patients' conditions do eventually deteriorate.

Vitamin E and anti-inflammatory drugs such as aspirin are being studied for their effectiveness in preventing and treating AD, with mixed results.

Herbal remedies such as ginkgo biloba are being studied also. But ginkgo biloba has a blood-thinning effect and can be dangerous when combined with other blood thinners, even common aspirin.

Reminder: Herbal remedies are medicine also. Always report any herbal remedy when your physician asks what medications you or your partner are taking.

A vaccine to block the beta-amyloid protein segment that forms plaques shows promise as a way to prevent and treat AD. Clinical trials on gene replacement therapy in human beings are under way.

Accepting the Diagnosis

Once you have a reliable diagnosis of your partner's dementia, it is important that *you* accept it. You must understand and work with your partner *the way the person is now.*

A good relationship with your partner depends on *you.* The person cannot be retaught. You cannot "reason" with him or her.

The person is not "just being difficult" or trying to "get back at you." Because the person cannot change, your approach toward him or her must change.

You are now the one in charge, the lead partner, and this may be a new role for you. Even if your partner appears normal most of the time, you *cannot* depend on him or her to use good judgment anymore. The person's safety and well-being depend on your acceptance of the caregiver's role.

Whether you tell your partner the diagnosis depends on his or her temperament and level of understanding. If the person is already very anxious or seems completely unaware of or denies symptoms, it may be best to avoid the subject. If the person asks, try saying "You are more forgetful than you used to be" or that he or she has "trouble with memory." See how this goes. If your partner responds well and asks for additional information, you can say more. If the person becomes extremely anxious and dwells on your remark, it would probably be better to stop there.

Accepting the diagnosis is essential to your relationship with your partner. Keep in mind that trying to make your partner relearn or remember things he or she has forgotten will not work. It will only upset the person and harm your relationship—your partnership. You will learn how to avoid or redirect your partner from difficult behaviors in this book, but you cannot make the person "better" or "normal."

Going On Together, Day by Day

Becoming and staying close—communicating naturally—is easier once you accept the diagnosis. It is the key to smoother sailing as a caregiver.

If you are new at this (an adult child now living with a parent or a sibling caring for a sibling, for example), you must get to know your relative better and learn to communicate effectively.

He or she will not be quite the same person you knew in the past. You will probably need to develop a different way of relating to the person.

It may become difficult to keep your relationship positive and to keep communicating well, even if you have been together a long time. You will now have to work at what used to come naturally. The method and nature of communication may need to change.

Suggestions: A person with mild dementia may be able to tell you how he or she feels and to understand what is happening. Many have written thoughtful accounts of what they experience. It is also very common, unfortunately, for a patient to deny that anything is wrong.

Regardless of your partner's awareness of the problem, set aside time each day to visit, observe your partner closely, and assess how he or she is doing. If your partner has severe dementia, the communication may be all nonverbal, but that is important too. You need to stay positive and receptive. The goal is to understand how your partner feels that day and to maintain your connection as the disease progresses. Pick a time with few distractions—a daily walk, afternoon tea, a drink before dinner, or drying dishes together.

You can't remember everything, so it helps considerably to keep some sort of an assessment diary. This could include notes on changes you see in your partner and how you deal with difficult situations. If your partner is able, his or her insights will help too. This diary will be useful at doctors' appointments and, most important, can guide you in understanding and dealing with your partner effectively as the disease progresses.

Daily talks and a diary will also be helpful if you are concerned about changes in your partner but are not sure there is a problem. They can help you (and your partner if he or she is aware of changes) decide if the patient needs an evaluation.

What if a difficult past cannot stay "in the past"? If your relationship with your family member was poor in the past, you need to decide if you can leave that history behind. Some issues can be put aside, some cannot. You need to be able to establish a close, positive relationship, or caregiving will be very difficult for you both. It is important to be honest with yourself and other family members. Sometimes a professional counselor can help. If your past together was very painful, it may be best for you to choose another caregiving option.

2 Preparing for the Future

Goal: This chapter will help you decide what long-term planning you need to do, both for your partner with dementia and for you.

Why Begin Long-Term Planning Now?

You may feel you can put off long-term planning if your partner's dementia is stable or is progressing very slowly. "Wait and see" is dangerous reasoning. If your partner suddenly declines more rapidly or exhibits behaviors that are too difficult for you to handle, you may need new legal, financial, or *long-term care* plans immediately.

You may feel you can wait because you are "in great shape" and "can handle anything." This can change without warning too, especially under the added stress of caregiving. Waiting could leave you and your partner in a precarious situation. Caregiving can be more stressful than you realize at the time.

Some words of caution:

- To stay in good health, make sure to spend time doing things that you enjoy and that have nothing to do with caregiving.

- Make time for plenty of rest and for your own physical care. Keep your doctor's appointments. You cannot be a good caregiver if you are tired, ill, or overly stressed.

If you are putting off long-term planning, examine your reasons. It is difficult, painful, and sad to plan the future for someone who has dementia. It is natural to want to put off such feelings for as long as possible. Putting them off may be another way of denying that there is a problem.

Try to keep in mind that you will feel more satisfied and less stressed once you are prepared. You will be better able to handle the future, even if it is very difficult. Reducing stress will also make you a better caregiver.

What Plans Do You Need to Make?

Make a list of things you know you need to do, questions, and concerns about long-term planning. Check it frequently, and revise it as needed. The clinic where your partner received the diagnosis of dementia should be able to advise you on long-term planning to some extent and to make referrals for you.

You need to start long-term planning now, but it will be an ongoing process and may change as your partner changes throughout the course of the disease. There are three main areas you will need to address:

1. establishing a good support system
2. health care planning
3. financial planning for you and your partner

Establishing a Good Support System

Involving Family Members and Friends: Usually but Not Always a Good Idea

You will probably need to inform other family members and per-haps close friends of the diagnosis when the time is appropriate. Close relatives may be hurt or angry if they are not informed, but deciding when to inform them is up to you and your partner. It may help you to share long-term planning concerns with at least some of them. Do not be embarrassed to state that a family mem-ber has dementia. Your life and your partner's will be easier if you don't try to hide it as symptoms become more severe.

As you go over your concerns and long-range planning ideas with family members, do not let them minimize your concerns. Their claim that "Dad's all right," for example, may make you want to back off and address issues later or "only if we need it." Your goal in involving your family is to gain new perspectives, helpful suggestions, and a good support system for yourself.

You might be surprised. Family members may offer assistance. Accept it if it is offered—you cannot do it all alone. They may have new ideas or even referrals for you. Responsible relatives can be the base for a good support system, but, if their involve-ment is in any way detrimental to you or your partner emotion-ally, don't hesitate to ask them to stay away.

Should the person with dementia be involved in these family discussions? Depending on your partner's level of understanding, he or she may be involved in informing others of the diagnosis. The person may also have other family members he or she con-fides in regularly. The patient needs a good support system too. Long-term planning, however, can be very frightening and diffi-cult for many ill people. It may be best to discuss plans for the future when your partner is elsewhere. If the person expresses concerns about the future, what he or she needs to hear is that you will be there for help and support. Do not make promises you may not be able to keep ("I will never place you in a nursing home" or "No one will ever care for you but me," for example).

Caring Professionals Can Help

There are literally hundreds of books and thousands of Web sites on AD and other dementias. There are several good dementia care journals, and conferences are held worldwide. There are also Internet chat rooms for caregivers—a support group whenever you need one.

The Alzheimer's Disease Education and Referral (ADEAR) Center is a service of the National Institute of Aging (NIH) and is an invaluable source of nationwide information. The Alzheimer's Association provides dementia-specific referrals, support groups, volunteer respite, caregiving training, and support. Check with your local office. (See Resources, page 129.)

Be very wary of caregiving Web sites and advertisements you know nothing about. There are many moneymaking scams touting far-fetched treatment, cures, and services. Speak to an aging or dementia specialist you trust to verify an organization's legitimacy.

Locate and Join a Good Support Group

Support groups are wonderful. Information from professionals is useful, but sharing concerns with others who face the same problems is often even more valuable. Not only are groups a great place to share ideas, but they also provide an opportunity to make new friends and get away from actual caregiving for a while. Remember Internet support groups also.

Support for your partner may be available. More and more attention is being paid to the specific, personal concerns of those with dementia. There may be a support group for those with de-

mentia in your area, and there is now a newsletter for those diagnosed with dementia: *Perspectives: A Newsletter for Individuals
with Alzheimer's Disease.*

Health Care Planning

Making Health Care Decisions for Your Partner

You will eventually need to take over health care decision making for your partner. You, or someone you trust, will need to have
a Durable Power of Attorney for Health Care (to be the agent)
or obtain conservatorship for your partner. You need to have appropriate long-term health care plans in place for yourself as well.

If you have already filled out a Durable Power of Attorney
form, examine it. If your partner with AD is listed as your agent,
be sure to change it. A person with dementia is, of course, *not* a
suitable agent.

The first thing on your health planning list should be Advance
Health Care Directives for both you and your partner. A directive
designates an agent and states long-term care and end-of-life
wishes. You do not need an attorney to execute this document,
but, if you have questions or there are problems, be sure to consult an attorney.

Depending on your partner's level of impairment, he or she
may still be able to execute a form. If your partner does not have
a directive and cannot or will not execute one, you or someone
you trust will need to be appointed conservator. If the person is
incapacitated but already has a directive with you or someone
you trust as Durable Power of Attorney for Health Care, you or
the other party should be able to take over health care management when needed.

You and your partner should both list alternate agents on your
forms. Choose your agent carefully. He or she must be older than
age eighteen and have no conflict of interest (be a long-term care

provider you use, for example). Your designated agent should be familiar with both your directive and your partner's. It is best if the agent lives nearby and knows where both forms are kept. This will ensure smooth transition of your partner's care if something happens to you.

Obtain a directive form from a notary, a health care agency, or the American Medical Association. They are also available online. You need a notary or two other people (not the agent) to witness the signing of the form.

Remember, the Advance Health Care Directive relates to care only. There is a separate Durable Power of Attorney for Finances. If you move from one state to another, you will need to execute a new directive in the new state. If you live part of the time in another state, you will need a Durable Power of Attorney in that state also.

Establishing a Conservatorship of Person

Conservatorship of person is done in a court, with an attorney present, so it can be very expensive. You will need to use it if your partner is too impaired to care for him- or herself but will not or cannot give you Durable Power of Attorney for Health Care. It is not the same as conservatorship of the estate.

A Lanterman-Petris-Short Act (LPS) conservatorship is one that is initiated by the court itself, under special circumstances and for very impaired individuals.

Choose Your Physician Carefully

Examine medical care for you and your partner. You need physicians who understand and support you and take the time to address your health care concerns. You may have known your primary care physicians for awhile, but, if they cannot provide the support you and/or your partner need now, don't be afraid to change. The important thing is that they be willing to spend the time you need by phone or by appointment. The advice they give must be sensitive to your individual needs and concerns. If it is not, try a recommendation from a health care professional or fellow caregiver you trust. Or call your health care group office or the local office of the American Medical Association for a referral. Look for a certified geriatrician (a physician specializing in the care of older adults) for primary care or a well-known neurologist or clinic for diagnostic services.

Be sure to read box 2-1, "Dealing Effectively with Physicians, Attorneys, and Other Professional Advisors."

Long-Term Care Options

Even if you feel you will never use long-term care, investigate the options now. You do not want to make a spur-of-the-moment, emergency decision. It is very important to check out the options, availability, and cost. Your financial planning must take into account the possibility of long-term care, including moving your partner to a full-time care facility. Unfortunately, most of them are expensive, so you will need to plan finances carefully.

It is a big step to admit that you need help with caregiving. Home care may be a good first choice, especially if you need only part-time assistance, because you maintain control of care to a greater extent and your partner will still be in your own home.

Long-term care agencies and communities specifically designed for those with dementia (such as adult day care, *assisted living, residential care,* and *skilled nursing* care settings) are a good choice for more extensive care because they are designed specifically to meet the needs of people with dementia. The type of long-term care which is best, however, is a decision for you and long-term care professionals to make together. All long-term care residential facilities have specific admission criteria that you will need to address. A mixed setting (in which residents with dementia and frail elderly residents share a facility) may be appropriate for some patients.

There are a number of long-term care options.

Family or volunteer respite. You are truly lucky if you have helpful family members. Some religious groups provide volunteer respite care providers.

Free government-funded in-home supportive services. These services may be available if your partner's income is low. They include assistance with basic daily living skills for only a few hours a week. If this care is available in your area, it is paid for and must be approved by the appropriate governmental body. The paid caregiver may be a family member.

Private home care. This includes a wide range of options, from occasional companion care to expensive full-time nursing. Medicare will pay for medically necessary short-term care by approved home health care agencies but not for long-term respite for a *chronic condition* such as dementia. Health insurance and long-term care insurance will pay for some in-home care. Be sure to investigate policies thoroughly. Long-term care management agencies are a relatively new care option. They supervise the overall care of a person for families who cannot do so themselves (for example, if the family lives out of the area). Make sure that your home liability coverage is adequate if you use in-home caregivers.

Home hospice care. This support service is paid for by Medicare for those who are terminally ill, and it provides valuable support for family members. Hospice care is also available in assisted living, residential, and skilled nursing facilities; hospice nurses and certified home health aides go there to provide end-of-life care.

Day care. Day care can be for mixed populations or specifically for those with dementia, frail elderly persons, or those with other specific diagnoses. It can be either social day care, some of which is dementia specific (usually regulated by the state's Department of Aging or state Community Care Licensing department), or adult day health care (usually regulated by the state's Department of Health Services). Adult day health care, along with other medical expenses, can be usually paid for by Medicaid, but social day care usually cannot. Long-term care insurance and the Veterans Administration may also pay for day care services.

Assisted living and residential care. Assisted living facilities are for larger communities that provide nonmedical help, such as assistance with dressing, bathing, and meals. An assisted living unit is a specific section of a retirement community. Assisted living can be Alzheimer specific, for frail older adults only, or for mixed populations. "Residential care" and "board and care" refer to smaller, homelike facilities. They have the same licensing requirements but usually have ten beds or fewer, and often an owner or manager lives on site. Both assisted living and residential care are regulated by special community care licensing agencies in most states and may or may not be paid for through Medicaid. If it specializes in dementia care or has even one resident with dementia, a board-and-care home must have approval from community care licensing agencies. Dementia care communities are often more expensive than mixed communities or those with no AD residents.

Skilled nursing care. Skilled nursing communities provide round-the-clock medical care, usually for persons with advanced dementia or with multiple problems. Skilled nursing is often the only option for low-income patients, however, because care can be paid for by Medicaid. Skilled nursing facilities are regulated by the state's Department of Health Services. Some are dementia specific or have special dementia care units, and some have mixed populations.

Financial Planning for You and Your Partner

Learn about Your Partner's Finances

It is often difficult to come to terms with the need to take over your partner's finances. It may feel very uncomfortable if this is a new role. In addition, someone with dementia can be paranoid about others looking into his or her financial affairs.

Understanding and organizing someone else's finances can be very complicated too. It may be even more difficult if the person has neglected financial matters or has used poor judgment due to dementia. On the other hand, if you have always managed finances as true partners, the task will be much easier.

Learn about your partner's complete economic situation: property, income, bills, and other debts and financial obligations.

Consult an Attorney

A good attorney is essential for making sound financial arrangements. Some attorneys specialize in elder law. The Alzheimer's Disease Education and Referral Center (ADEAR) or the Alzheimer's Association may be able to give you good referrals. You can also contact the local chapter of the Bar Association. The attorney should offer a complimentary first visit. If you have not yet consulted with an attorney in regard to your new situation as a caregiver, do so immediately.

Design an Appropriate, Detailed Long-Term Financial Plan

Developing a long-term financial plan is a time-consuming process. You will need to arrange for the management of day-to-day financial obligations, property, and investments. Some procedures used to transfer responsibility for financial assets are Durable Power of Attorney for Asset Management, Revocable Living Trusts, and Conservatorship of the Estate.

You will also have to develop long-term care choices that are suitable for your partner. Make choices based on the financial assets available. Remember, you must plan for what may happen in the future, not just the current situation. Determine methods for payment of long-term care now—don't wait. Remember to check into health and long-term care insurance benefits. The Veterans Administration may provide assistance if your partner is a veteran. Look at Supplemental Social Security benefits, long-term care tax credits, and in-home supportive services in addition to Medicaid if the patient's income is low.

Protect Your Own Financial Stability

With your attorney try to establish financial arrangements that will not deplete your personal assets too severely but will still allow your partner to live comfortably and safely throughout the course of the dementia. You must be careful not to deplete your own resources too much if the person with dementia has little or no money of his or her own. Your attorney and long-term care advisors can help you decide on the best financial arrangements. Keep in mind your other financial responsibilities. Not only must you care for your partner, but you must also maintain your own financial stability and that of any other dependent family members.

If you are a spouse, assets you hold alone are not at risk, but Medicaid will not help with your partner's long-term care and other medical expenses until you spend some joint assets. You will be able to retain your home, car, and certain cash reserves and investments. You must consult an attorney. There are many ways to protect your fair share of your assets. You do not need to become impoverished to get help with your partner's care. For example, you might have made promises to a parent or spouse in regard to long-term care which are difficult to keep when you are confronted with the realities of dementia care.

Loretta and her husband, Anthony, had promised each other that they would stay close and take care of each other until they died. As Anthony's Alzheimer disease worsened, however, he became very agitated and often did not recognize Loretta. When he didn't, he would often order her out of the house, and he even called the police a few times. When he took medication for his anxiety and delusions, he became very lethargic, and she was unable to give him enough assistance with his daily tasks such as dressing and bathing. Her son came and helped as often as possible, but he lived in another city, worked full-time, and had his own family responsibilities.

Loretta became very depressed. A friend suggested a large assisted living facility nearby, but it was expensive, and Loretta felt she would be breaking her promise to Anthony if she placed him there. An additional problem with placement was that, though she had enough money to live on, she calculated that she would eventually have to dip deeply into savings and might have to sell her home to keep him there. (Remember, Medicaid will not pay for assisted living.)

Loretta also had an ill sister who lived far away, and Loretta wanted to go see her a few times while she was still able to enjoy visits. These visits were an additional expense that she could not afford if she placed Anthony in the facility, but what would she do with Anthony while she was gone? She tried leaving him with her son twice, but Anthony became extremely upset and tried to leave. It frightened the grandchildren, and Loretta did not want them to have unpleasant or frightening memories of their grandfather.

In long talks with her son Loretta finally agreed that neither she nor her husband had expected an illness like Alzheimer disease and that it was not safe for either her or Anthony for him to remain home with her anymore. She and her son consulted a financial advisor and arranged her finances so that she could have enough to live on and keep her home if she placed him in a smaller and much more modest board-and-care home. She transferred some assets to her name only and arranged for her son to be conservator for her husband. She trusted her son's judgment and knew he would consult with her on all decisions. The conservatorship relieved her mind of the worry about what would happen to Anthony if she became ill and relieved her of the strain of sole responsibility.

Loretta felt she kept her promise to Anthony, at least in part, by visiting him at least twice a week and by taking him on outings that were fun for both of them. She also made unannounced visits to keep a close eye on the care Anthony was receiving. Her financial arrangements left her with enough money to visit her sister several more times, even though she had to live more modestly in other ways. Her son made sure he visited his father more frequently while she was away on these visits.

Pay attention to the details when consulting professional advisors (see box 2-1). There are agencies and other sources that will help you with your planning and will provide you with good support:

- local and state aging services departments
- the Alzheimer's Association (local and national)
- local adult day care and residential care settings specializing in dementia care
- books, journals, Web sites, and national associations such as the American Society on Aging

Box 2-1. Dealing Effectively with Attorneys, Physicians, and Other Professional Advisors

When you work with professional advisors, you need to be well prepared. Here are steps you should *always* take:

1. Write down all information during any important phone calls—names of those to whom you speak, spelling of names, job titles, addresses, phone numbers, dates and times of calls, and summaries of the conversations. Use a log you can keep for reference, not just the closest sheet of paper! Also, keep with the log any correspondence related to the matters you are investigating.

2. When making an appointment, inform the office if you will need to ask a lot of questions during the visit. They can then allocate time accordingly.

3. Ahead of time, write out questions you need to ask.

4. Ahead of time, assemble any documents or other material you will need.

5. Begin an appointment with a brief overview of the reason for your visit or call. Try not to get off topic. Keep questions short and to the point.

6. At an appointment, write down instructions you receive and responses to your questions. Also, repeat important information back to the person you are conferring with, asking whether you understood correctly. Don't rely on memory for later recall—perfect recollection is never possible, even though we sometimes like to think it is!

7. Let the physician know ahead of time if you have questions you are uncomfortable asking in front of your partner. You can request a telephone appointment or see the physician separately. You can even provide a written statement of your questions or concerns ahead of time.

You Can Still Look Forward to the Future

Do not give up on those retirement plans or special events you have been thinking about for years. The future may need to be different from what you had planned but can still create good memories.

If your partner is still only mildly impaired, do the things you want to do now. For example, if you always wanted to retire to a place in the mountains, rent first instead of buying and see how you both adjust. If you wait until later, a move might be impossible.

You will probably need to adapt your plans as the dementia progresses, but you may not need to cancel plans completely. Simplify, use "trial runs," or perhaps get additional help.

Simplify special events. For example, invite just a few guests to a fiftieth wedding anniversary party. Try it earlier in the day and for a shorter period. Perhaps you can have refreshments and dancing or dinner only rather than both dinner and dancing.

Not sure if an event is a good idea? Try a short trial run before the big event. For example, try a two-day cruise before trying a long one. Simplify your life on board the ship too. Perhaps avoid the late-night parties and many of the off-ship excursions.

Try bringing along a third person or an understanding second couple on that cruise or another type of vacation. Then you will have help if needed and occasional respite from caregiving.

3 Communication, the Key to Quality of Life for You and Your Loved One

Goal: This chapter will equip you with the tools you need for positive interaction with your partner and for effectively managing difficult behaviors (including *catastrophic reactions*).

What Is Dementia Like?

What is it like to have dementia? How does it feel when you can't understand what others are telling you? It must feel as though you are continually in a new situation, trying to figure out what is going on.

Try an experiment. Turn a novel to a page somewhere in the middle and read a couple of pages. Do you understand who is who and why things are happening as they are? It is probably confusing. Your partner feels this way every day. Just as you need to start from the beginning of the book to fill in the blanks, your partner depends on you to fill in the blanks for him or her. This dependence on you is why so many persons with dementia have "separation anxiety" when you leave them. You are their lifeline—quite a burden for you but so important to them.

Positive Interaction Techniques

Interaction is two-way communication. It is the process of using verbal language and nonverbal language such as facial expression and body language to send and receive messages. To communicate with your partner effectively, you need to suit your communication methods to the person's mood, degree of attention, and general ability to function at that particular moment.

We think of spoken and written (verbal) language as our primary method of communication, but 90 percent of all interaction is nonverbal. Think about how important nonverbal communication is to your partner with AD. The patient's problems with communication result from some of the (PALMER) symptoms he or she is experiencing—short attention span and impaired language, memory, and reasoning and judgment skills—and you must adapt your communication techniques so that the person understands you despite these debilitating symptoms.

The use of *positive interaction techniques* will not only help you and your partner understand each other better but will also, it is hoped, make your life together a more pleasant experience.

The Basics of Positive Interaction Techniques

Positive interaction techniques are the key to success with your partner. As a patient loses the ability to communicate with words, he or she may still understand some or even much of what you are saying and how you are feeling by reading nonverbal cues.

- The person will probably act angry, sad, or upset when you appear angry, sad, or upset—just when you can least cope with it. This is called "mirroring."
- To gain positive results, you will need to try to act calm and relaxed (the way you want your partner to act) all of the time, even when you do not feel like it.

Box 3-1. Four Basic Rules for Positive Interactions

1. Stay pleasant, calm, and reassuring to help keep your partner feeling that way.
2. Always help your partner maintain positive self-esteem.
3. Help your partner understand you by using simple sentences and repeating them as needed.
4. Help your partner understand by using nonverbal cues.

One of the difficult things about dementia for you is losing the support and encouragement of your partner, the very things that make a partnership.

Four Basic Rules for Positive Interactions (box 3-1)

1. Stay Pleasant, Calm, and Reassuring to Keep the Person That Way

Be aware of your voice. Tone, pitch, speed of speech, and inflection are all important. Your tone should be soothing and sound pleasant, especially if your partner is upset or angry. Keep the pitch somewhere in the middle. High-pitched voices can be jarring to the nerves; a low pitch can seem threatening. Moderate the speed of your speech. If your speech is too slow, the person may lose the thread of what you are saying; if it is too fast, he or she may not be able to follow. *Inflection* helps the person understand the meaning of what you are saying. Be very aware of it. Make sure that it helps him or her understand what you are trying to convey.

Be aware of the message given by your body language. Keep your face relaxed and smiling. Your eyes need to look that way too. It is hard to keep your features calm and pleasant if you do not feel that way, but your partner will read your face and become upset if you do not look pleasant, calm, and reassuring. Be aware of your body posture and your hand and arm movements. Lean forward and open your hands and arms. Leaning back, folded arms, arms tight against the body, and clenched fists all convey a negative message.

Make sure that what is going on in the physical environment around the person is also relaxing and serene.

2. Always Help the Person Maintain Positive Self-Esteem

Think of and treat your partner as your equal, all the time, regardless of his or her behavior at the moment. This is called "unconditional positive regard." Avoid negatives ("Don't do that!") or criticism ("You look terrible in that old shirt!").

Never talk about your partner in front of him or her, and don't let others do so. This is hard because it may often seem as though your partner is mentally far, far away. It also is easier to talk right where you are than to move. You may not even realize that you are doing it. Even an affectionate home care aide or your physician may make this mistake. If others are discussing your partner in his or her presence, deliberately and obviously include your partner in the conversation or ask the other person to wait a minute and guide him or her off to one side to talk. Be sure to talk to the person who was speaking in front of your partner about it later to reduce the risk of it happening again.

Never use "baby talk" (for example, using the phrase "go potty") and avoid a condescending tone of voice. This can be very embarrassing for the patient. Again, you may not be aware of it, so be careful, and do not let others do it either. If there are terms of endearment you both use or a childhood phrase works to get the message across, however, then it is okay. Just don't use such terms when it is unnecessary.

Avoid "why" questions (for example, "Why did you put mashed potatoes in your coffee instead of the cream?"). Your partner will feel flustered and embarrassed and cannot tell you why.

Remember that basic symptom, lack of reasoning and judgment: your partner cannot be expected to explain his or her actions.

Let the person be as independent as he or she can safely be. Give the patient choices whenever possible (also see chaps. 5 and 6). For example, if he or she cannot choose clothing independently, hold up two shirts and ask, "Would you like to wear the blue one or the yellow one?" If the person cannot choose, try, "I think you would look wonderful in the yellow shirt." You are really not giving the person a choice, but it is offered as a suggestion, not an order.

3. Help the Person Understand by Using Simple Sentences and by Repeating as Needed

Caution: Communication is important to every human being. Speak to mildly impaired patients as normally as possible. They will be offended if you simplify ideas and sentences too much. At the other extreme, even the best communication techniques may not work with very impaired patients. The act of communicating, however, is important to both of them.

Use simple sentences. Remember that mildly impaired patients need less simplification. For patients with moderate and severe impairment, use simple sentences and repeat them as needed. For example, one idea and one *step* is "Joe, sit down." "Joe, pick up the photo album and come and sit down with me" is two ideas and two steps. A step is an action complete in itself. It doesn't require memory of other steps to complete it.

Repeat as needed. It may take more than once for your partner to understand an idea or instruction from you. You may need to repeat it several times. If it is an instruction for a task, repeat it as the person does it, so the person does not forget what he or she is doing. Remember that basic symptom, a short attention span. When repeating, if your partner doesn't understand you after a couple of tries, choose a different phrase. For example, if he or she doesn't understand "It's time for lunch" after a couple of repeats, say, "Come and eat a sandwich," or another phrase your partner might understand better.

4. Help the Person Understand by Using Nonverbal Cues

Remember the importance of using good body language. Also use eye contact. First, get and maintain eye contact. Then, if you're helping your partner undertake a task, show the person the objects involved to help him or her understand. Make sure your partner first sees you and then sees what you are holding, pointing at, or touching. Look at the person's eyes to see if he or she really sees and understands. There is a difference between just looking at something and looking at it with understanding.

When you need to guide them somewhere, very impaired loved ones may respond best if you stand facing them, grasp both of their hands gently, and pull them forward, keeping eye contact, as you walk backward toward where you need to go. For example, if it is time for lunch, try standing in front of your partner, look into his or her eyes, and say, "Hi. It's time for lunch." When you can tell from the person's eyes that he or she sees you, show the lunch plate and say, "It's time for lunch." When you see the person look at the plate, repeat that it is time for lunch. Then say, "Sit down to eat," pointing to the table and tapping the chair. When the person sees and understands, guide him or her, by both hands if necessary, to sit down.

Use all the senses to give cues: visual, olfactory, auditory, and tactile. If your partner is mildly or even moderately impaired, he or she will probably not need as many cues as someone who is severely impaired. It is important not to help too much. This can create what is called an *excess disability* (see also chaps. 5 and 6). No matter how hard you try, it may be very difficult to communicate with a severely impaired partner. It may be difficult to understand the person's verbal and nonverbal communication correctly.

If you can't understand your partner, try not to let your frustration show because this may upset him or her and make communication even more difficult. Try to put yourself in the person's shoes and figure out how you would feel if your loved ones could not understand you. This is empathy. Give the person a hug; tell your partner you love him or her. Show your sympathy, interest, and support. This is validation. Don't ignore him or her or walk away. If you just nod, even if you don't understand, you are acknowledging the person's importance and need to communicate. Communication is a basic need of all human beings.

The person may use nonsense words or be nonverbal. The person may mutter to him- or herself and look down most of the time, not at others. If this is true for your partner, try to figure out what the person wants or needs by observing nonverbal cues, such as body language and facial expressions.

The person may say the same word or phrase over and over (perseveration). He or she may be "stuck" on the word and be unable to get past it or may be just vocalizing. Try giving the person a "jump start": say the word the person says, and then pause. The person may then be able to complete the thought. Also look at nonverbal cues: where the person is looking, his or her facial expression, body language, and actions.

Bob's father, Harry, had slowly lost most of his language skills with the progression of dementia. He would try to tell Bob something and be unable to say the word he wanted, would get frustrated, and then would have even more trouble speaking. He had the most trouble with nouns and adjectives—the specific names of and descriptive words for everyday things. When Bob was helping him dress, he would tell Bob he wanted to put on his _____ and lose the words. Or, for some reason, he would use the word brown to fill in the blank for any word he could not say. For example, he might say, "I want to put on my _____ brown." If he gestured to his upper torso, Bob would fill in the statement with "your shirt." He would then guide Harry to the closet, pick a shirt, show it to him, and say, "What about this one?"

Harry still maintained very definite preferences and would either agree with Bob's choice or shake his head and point to another one.

Bob knew to allow extra time for dressing and other tasks. But when time was short for dressing, he would get the appropriate clothes and just say, "This will look great on you, Dad." He would make sure Harry was looking right at him, that he saw his warm facial expression and smile, heard his calm tone of voice, and actually saw the garment. He would accompany the instructions with a hug or gentle shoulder rub. This usually worked because Harry interpreted Bob's actions as meaning he was not angry or impatient, just making a suggestion.

Managing Difficult Behaviors

Some patients with dementia stay calm and unruffled throughout the disease process, but, unfortunately, these folks are few and far between. You need to "be a detective" to deal effectively with difficult behaviors common to dementia.

Keep in mind that you cannot make your partner behave normally again, but you can often make difficult behaviors easier to live with. Adjust your expectations to suit the person's level of disability and "pick your battles." There are behaviors you may not be able to modify.

By being a detective, we mean doing ongoing assessment. You must look at external, internal, and "invisible" causes of your partner's behavior. External causes are things that have happened or are happening around or to the person. Internal causes are discomfort and pain caused by illness, living habits, or injury. Invisible causes are declines in functioning due to the disease process or misinterpretations of what is going on around the person, such as *hallucinations* and *delusions*. Empathy is important. If you try to put yourself in the person's shoes, it may be easier for you to understand a problem and, it is hoped, improve the situation.

You must change your perception of what constitutes correct behavior for your partner. This behavior is normal for someone with dementia. The changes in the brain cannot be reversed, and your partner's behavior is beyond his or her control. All the behaviors have reasons, but they may be difficult for you to determine. Remember: this is not the person's "second childhood." The person behaves this way because he or she has a disability.

Some Difficult Behaviors Common in Dementia (box 3-2)

It is impossible to address all the problem behaviors individually in one chapter, but we hope the techniques given here will help you. Remember that your situation in coping with these behaviors is not unique. You can learn how to deal with them from fellow caregivers in support groups or read books specifically on managing difficult behaviors.

Always remember that you can only do your best, and dealing with difficult behaviors is a very hard job.

A Behavior Management Tool

A detective looks at all aspects of a case: who, what, when, where, why, and how. This is what you need to do to try and manage a behavior problem (box 3-3).

Decide If It Really Is a Problem

Some behaviors are easier to live with than to challenge. Determine:

- Is it harmful to you or to your partner?
- Does it keep your partner from doing other things that might satisfy him or her more, given the stage of dementia?
- Does it keep you from doing things you must do for your safety

---

Box 3-2. Common Behavior Problems

- Anxiety
- Confusing day and night
- Paranoia and suspicion
- Wandering and pacing
- Refusal to eat
- Eating nonfood items
- Depression
- Hoarding: collecting and keeping items from others
- Sexually inappropriate behaviors
- Gulping or hoarding food
- Apathy: disinterest, lack of motivation for activity
- Poor grooming, dressing, and bathing habits
- Outbursts: emotional, verbal, physical aggression
- Repetitive behaviors: actions, words, or ideas
- Rummaging: looking through and moving about objects, drawers, cabinets, closets, or boxes
- Inappropriate social behaviors: undressing in public, inappropriate conversation with others
- Inappropriate toileting habits: use of containers other than the toilet or urinating or defecating in public

---

and health and your partner's, or does it keep you from functioning well, physically and emotionally?

Barbara's brother Arthur insists on wearing the same yellow shirt every day. He becomes very worried and upset if he is unable to wear it. It disturbs Barbara because he used to be so careful about his dress and has a closet full of perfectly good shirts. The yellow shirt is fairly new, however, and looks good enough to wear out in public as well as around the house.

Box 3-3. How to Analyze and Manage a Problem Behavior

Decide:

1. Is it really a problem?
2. What is the problem?
3. With whom does it occur—just you, or specific other people?
4. Where does it occur—anywhere? away from home? some specific place in the house? the yard?
5. When does it occur—any particular time of day?

Then:

6. Try to figure out why it is occurring.
7. Consider how you are going to manage it.
8. Decide on a course of action.
9. Stick to it for at least a couple of days. Make sure anyone else providing care tries it, too. (It needs more than one try to see if it may be successful.)
10. Analyze the situation again.
11. If necessary, try another solution.

Arthur's insistence on wearing his yellow shirt is not a problem because wearing the shirt does not keep him from doing other things. It does not harm or disrupt Barbara's life in any way (unless she lets it upset her), and it certainly does not hurt anyone else.

Approaches Barbara could use: She could resign herself to the one shirt. She could buy him several more just like it and let him put one on every day.

General approaches:

- If it is not a problem, take a deep breath and remind yourself, again, that you must redefine your idea of success and pick your battles.

- If it is a problem, proceed with the steps outlined next and try to make the situation better.

Decide What the Problem Is

There may really be several different problems. If you figure out what the root problem is and do something about it, the others may diminish or even disappear.

Maria's husband with AD loves to be outside but tramples the flowers and vegetables in her garden because he does not seem to be aware that they are there.

The basic problem is not that he tramples the garden but that he paces. If Maria addresses the root problem, pacing, the garden problem will diminish or disappear.

Approaches Maria could use: Pacing is not a problem in itself. Maria needs to create a different place for her husband to pace, away from the garden.

General approaches:

- Study the problem for a couple of days. Take notes on it in your caregiver diary (see chap. 1). Perhaps get a friend or relative to look at the situation with you for a different perspective.
- Sometimes you cannot figure out the root problem in a complex situation. It is then a matter of trying different approaches one by one.

With Whom Does the Problem Occur?

Does the problem occur only with you, only when others are around, or only when other specific people are present?

Harvey's wife sticks close by him all day. She insists on staying in the same room or the same section of the yard. She enjoys visits from her female friends but is very uneasy with Harvey's male friends and sticks to him "like glue" when they are there. Harvey looks forward to these visits but cannot enjoy them when his wife stays so close.

The problem is that Harvey's wife is uncomfortable around men other than her husband.

Approaches Harvey could use: Once he figures out that it is specifically men who bother his wife, Harvey is prepared for it and handles it better. He gets his daughter to come by occasionally, she takes his wife into another room, and Harvey then slips out to visit with "the boys" elsewhere.

General approaches:

- Once you figure out with whom the problem occurs, work around it.
- Additional caution: Anytime your partner has unusually negative reactions to a new caregiver, whether it be a paid caregiver, friend, or family member, be concerned. Observe them together for awhile. In addition, leave for a short time while the new caregiver is there and then arrive home unexpectedly. This new caregiver may be using inappropriate interaction techniques or may even be abusing your partner, verbally or physically. Check for skin tears or bruising. It may be difficult for you, but you must deal with it. Remember, your partner will probably not be able to tell you much about problems. You must observe, assess, and determine how to deal with the situation.

Where Does the Problem Occur?

The physical environment affects behavior. Remember, it must be calm, pleasant, and reassuring. Your partner may have fewer behavior problems in certain parts of the house. Large open areas (a room with a cathedral ceiling, for example) may bother him or her. The person probably feels less protected there. Problems occur in unfamiliar settings but also when a person is cooped up in the same area for too long.

Mrs. Sparks used to love gardening, but her dementia is now more severe. Mr. Sparks is concerned because she refuses to join him in the garden, and he is afraid to leave her alone in the house.

The problems are:

- Mrs. Sparks is afraid of the outdoors because she feels exposed and unprotected there.
- She may also feel like she is far away from home when she's outside. People with dementia commonly react this way to open areas.
- Glare or low light, wind, and temperature differences can increase the sense of being in a strange place.

Approaches Mr. Sparks could try: He can highlight the door to the house, paint the edges a bright color, or put colorful plants along each side so Mrs. Sparks can see the door more clearly.

Mr. Sparks can point to the door and reassure her that she is not far from home. If this does not work, he could try installing an awning over a patio just outside the back door. She could stay there while he gardened. Mrs. Sparks would still feel protected by a roof, and it would reduce glare and wind.

General approaches: Your partner cannot understand and adjust to an environment that is distressing him or her for some reason. You must change it, whenever possible, to suit the person. Environmental problems are easier to manage than others, because they are something real and concrete which you can usually modify to some extent for comfort.

When Does the Problem Occur?

Patients have more behavior problems when they are tired. There-fore, they tend to have fewer problems in the morning and more later in the day. This tendency to have problems late in the day is called *sundowning*. Sundowning is usually expressed as anxi-ety, restlessness, or refusal to do anything. It is also common for a person to want to "go home," even if he or she is already home. Night and day reversals are also a problem.

Paul's mother was always alert and happy in the morning and took her baths then. She suddenly began resisting and finally refused to bathe. He noticed that she had dark circles under her eyes, and he checked her to see if she was ill. She had no fever or other symptoms, so he decided to check on her more at night.

The problem turned out to be that she was rummaging through her drawers most of the night, was not sleeping, and was therefore too tired to bathe in the morning.

Approaches Paul could try: He should assess his mother's rou-tine. Is something keeping her awake (a change in the household routine—noise, activity, or too much light at night)? Is she drink-ing water or caffeine at night? Is she sleeping during the day? If there are no changes in the routine, he will need to have her ex-amined by her physician. She may be ill, or the physician may need to adjust medications or prescribe something to help her sleep.

General approaches: Assess the routine and adjust it to suit your partner as much as possible. See a physician if the prob-lem persists. If the problem is sundowning, keep the routine dur-ing the problem time consistent, do not expect the person to do difficult or stressful tasks, and keep reassuring him or her that everything is okay. Soothing music and easy activities they enjoy will help many patients. It is usually worse if they have nothing to do.

Why Some Behavior Problems Occur and How They Can Be Managed

This section looks at common causes for some behavior problems and general hints on how you can manage them. These hints may help you avoid some problems in the first place.

Physical Problem as a Cause

Look to a physical condition (discomfort, pain, or illness) as a cause of a behavior before looking at any other causes. The best clues that your partner may be in physical distress are a general reduction in ability to function, a new difficult behavior, or an increase in severity of an existing behavior. For example, a sudden increase in the general level of confusion is often the first symptom of a urinary tract infection or pneumonia.

If you can relieve the discomfort, pain, or illness, the behavior may be avoided or go away. Discomfort can be caused by little things you could handle easily but your partner cannot. For example, could the person be dehydrated or hungry? Are the hearing aids or dentures in place, and do they fit well? Does the person need to go to the bathroom?

If you even suspect a problem with pain or illness, contact your physician immediately. You need to check on the person's physical condition daily because he or she probably cannot tell you when something is wrong.

Signs of discomfort or pain include fidgeting, pulling at clothing, change in body posture or gait, reduced attention span, rubbing a specific part of the body, a tense or worried facial expression, refusal to move about or do usual activities, limping, and holding or protecting specific body parts.

Signs of illness can include the usual symptoms of cold or flu, including vomiting, diarrhea, and fever. (Older adults' normal body temperature is usually a little below ninety-eight degrees.) Also look for pale, bluish, or dry lips and cold, clammy, or elastic skin (skin can become loose when it is dehydrated). Other symptoms can include refusal to eat or drink, a change in bowel or bladder habits (including *incontinence*), swelling, rash, rapid breathing, coughing, gasping for breath, a change in heart rate or pulse, an increase in hallucinations and delusions, and loss of general awareness or consciousness.

Medication as a Cause

Suspect medication as a cause if there is loss of awareness or consciousness, drowsiness, problems with *ambulation* (including dizziness), change in gait, inability to control body movements (ataxia), constipation, incontinence, rash, or reduction in blood pressure. Work with your physician to manage the problem—never alone!

Additional important points about medications, your partner's and yours:

- Make sure your physicians know about all medications you or your partner are taking, including over-the-counter medications, herbal remedies, and prescriptions.
- Report any change for the worse to the physician immediately.
- Remember that some side effects can probably be expected, especially in frail elderly persons. Ask the physician what to expect, what is "normal."
- Request the smallest possible dosage first; see the physician again if it seems inaccurate.
- Allow at least two weeks for a medication to take effect, but, of course, report any change in your partner's condition for the worse immediately.
- Be very careful to stick to the recommended dosage. In addition, never stop a medication without first consulting your physician.

- Never let your partner take medication unsupervised. This is important even with mildly impaired patients because taking too little or too much can have dire consequences.
- Be aware that generic medications may affect you or your partner differently from a name brand. Many health plans have a specific list of medications (called a *formulary*) from which your physician can choose. Remember, any time a medication does not have the result you expect, check with your physician. If a generic medication does not work for you, your physician can usually authorize a brand name medication. Be particularly cautious if you are used to a name brand and are switched to a generic.

Other Common Causes of Difficult Behavior

Hallucinations and Delusions

It is important not to tell your partner he or she is wrong or deny what the person is experiencing. Hallucinations or delusions are very real to him or her. If you deny that they are real, the person may become upset and afraid to trust you. Simply reassure the person, several times if needed. Tell the person that you will take care of it but don't elaborate. You do not want to make the problem more elaborate and intense than it already is.

For example, if your partner sees a strange man in the corner (a hallucination), do not just say, "Go away." Simply assure your partner that you will take care of it, guide the person away from that area, and try to distract him or her toward something else.

A Problem Communicating

Use positive interaction techniques. Remember to simplify and use multiple *sensory* cues.

An Uncomfortable or Upsetting Physical Environment

(See "Where Does the Problem Occur?" on p. 47)

Fatigue or Day/Night Reversal

(See "When Does the Problem Occur?" on p. 49)

Activities That Are Too Difficult or Too Easy or If Your Partner Has Too Much or Not Enough to Do

Excess disability can be caused by too many demands or not enough. Both are detrimental, and both can result in difficult behaviors because your partner is embarrassed, frustrated, or just not interested in what is being asked of him or her. Never force your partner to do something! This may cause a catastrophic reaction.

Reassess and adjust the tasks and methods you use accordingly. Try to stick to a set routine each day but be flexible within the routine. For example:

- Have breakfast, lunch, dinner, and walks at the same time daily, but, if family or friends come by or it is pouring rain, don't be afraid to be flexible.
- If your partner is enjoying a football game on television, postpone your usual walk until later.

Inability to Do Once-Familiar Tasks

The inability to do once-familiar tasks can cause your partner to feel frustrated and inadequate. The person may also feel that you are deliberately keeping him or her from doing the activity and become very angry. Examples are handling money, balancing the checkbook, or taking a walk alone. Such problems are difficult to manage and require creativity on your part. One of the worst problems is driving because it is very dangerous for a person diagnosed with dementia to drive. Your partner may insist on driving and become angry with you when you refuse to let him or her do so.

If you have only one car:

- Get a prescription from your physician which you can show your partner stipulating no driving.
- Get a note from your insurance company (on its stationery) stipulating no driving.
- Hide the car keys or have an antitheft chip installed, so only you can turn on the car.
- If your partner becomes upset while you are driving (arguing, trying to get out, grabbing the wheel), you may need to avoid traveling with him or her alone. Use taxis or have a friend drive, with you and your partner in back.

If you have two cars:

- Get a statement on insurance company stationery to show to your partner which states that you are the sole driver for both cars.
- Disable your partner's car, stating that it cannot be fixed.
- Remove your partner's car from the garage. Out of sight, out of mind!

Difficulty Stopping an Activity (Perseveration) Causing Difficult Behavior

If your partner has trouble ending an activity, try to attract the person's attention. Guide the person away from the activity by using alternatives he or she enjoys (use visual cues, for instance, a cookie or other favorite snack) or try to remove supplies, if applicable. The idea is to redirect the person.

Disorientation Due to Poor Memory and Perceptual Problems

Disorientation can cause wandering and be a severe problem. More than 60 percent of persons with AD wander off at some point. Try to educate friends and neighbors who live nearby in case you need their help.

Keep a cell phone handy in case your partner bolts from the

house and you must follow. Make sure the phone numbers for police, friends, and relatives who can help are coded onto or near your cell phone and home phone.

You may want to get cards that state: "The person with me has Alzheimer disease (or dementia). I need help. Please call the police. The number for the police department is _____." You can give them to people you encounter if your partner bolts and you need to follow.

Most important: Register with the Alzheimer's Association Safe Return Program. It is a low-cost nationwide data base that identifies individuals with dementia through a bracelet inscribed with a personal ID code; scholarships are also available. (For information nationwide, call 888-572-8566, or call your local Alzheimer's Association office.)

Catastrophic Reactions

Avoiding a catastrophic reaction (box 3-4) is, of course, easier than actually having to deal with one. Communicating with and assessing your partner frequently is the key. If you see your partner frowning, looking anxious, or wringing his or her hands, don't just wait to see what happens. Try to manage the situation before it gets any worse.

There are some precautions you can take before a catastrophic reaction happens:

- Remember to store soothing things your partner enjoys where you can access them easily.
- Refer to the section on wandering.

The causes of catastrophic reactions are the same as those for behavior problems. The difference is that a catastrophic reaction is a sudden change for the worse which can quickly become very difficult or even impossible to manage (box 3-5).

Box 3-4. Catastrophic Reactions

A catastrophic reaction is any sudden change in behavior for the worse, such as:
- verbal or physical aggression
- worry
- anger
- tension in the body or in facial expression
- rapid mood change
- stubborn resistance
- pacing or wandering
- paranoia
- crying
- hysterical laughter
- sudden self-isolation, refusal to speak

Remember, all behavior has a reason. It is a response to external, internal, or invisible stimuli. But you handle a catastrophic reaction differently from a behavior problem. With a catastrophic reaction you take specific steps immediately to make the situation manageable and then think about it later, to keep it from happening again. The immediate well-being and safety of both you and your partner is your prime concern. With a behavior problem you need to be the detective and determine causes as you try for a solution. A behavior problem can be managed gradually because it is not an immediate, serious, dangerous, or potentially dangerous situation.

Bea's husband, Theo, is moderately impaired but becomes extremely anxious and even angry if he cannot concentrate on things he used to be able to do with ease. The city was repairing the road in front of

Box 3-5. What to Do If a Catastrophic Reaction Occurs

1. Reassure your partner ("Everything will be okay; it's all right"). Make sure you act, look, and sound relaxed and calm (positive interaction techniques). Caution: If the person is very angry, reassure from a distance.

2. Reduce all outside stimulation and hazards. Stimulation includes loud music, a barking dog, children running or playing close by, the dishwasher running, the television, or anything else that could be irritating. Remember the importance of having a calm, pleasant, and reassuring environment. Remove objects that could cause harm, such as scissors or hot coffee.

3. If reducing stimulation and removing hazards is not feasible, remove your partner. For example, if the dog barking bothers your partner, close the window or try to mask the sound with soft music. If that doesn't help, take your partner to another area of the house. Don't try to force your partner to move, however, as he or she will only become more upset. Stay calm, pleasant, and reassuring.

4. Reassure again. Try touch now if your partner was too upset to approach before. Don't get too close if the person is still very angry.

5. Redirect to an easy, soothing activity in a quiet area. This does not mean a card game or anything too challenging or stimulating. It might be quiet, soothing music. Sing or hum along. You might try holding hands or giving your partner a neck rub. Looking at a favorite photo album or eating a favorite cookie might be good. Note: Think about putting some of your partner's favorite soothing things in a spot easy for you to get to "just in case" a catastrophic reaction takes place.

6. Be patient. Waiting for a catastrophic reaction to stop can seem like forever.

(continued)

**Box 3-5. What to Do If a Catastrophic
Reaction Occurs** *(continued)*

7. If you cannot stop it or if the person's anger is directed at you, leave your partner alone if it is safe (remember to remove hazardous objects). "Alone" means ten feet away or in a corner so you are inconspicuous (someplace where you can see your partner but he or she cannot see you is best). You do not want to become part of the problem or a greater part of the problem. If you try to stay too close by, try to soothe your partner when he or she is not ready, or try to argue, the person's anger may be redirected toward you or may increase toward you.

8. When your partner is calmer, return as if nothing has happened. Don't ask, "Why were you angry?" or "Why did you yell at me?" It hurts when you are trying to do your best and your partner lashes out at you. Remember, however, it is the disease talking. Your partner cannot help it and may not even remember the incident afterward.

9. After it is over, you need to think about the incident. It is probably the last thing in the world you want to think about again, but it is necessary. Remember, common causes of catastrophic reactions are the same as those for behavior problems. They are just sudden, more severe reactions. Perhaps take notes in your caregiver notebook. Try to think it through to see whether there is anything you can do to try to keep it from happening again.

---

the house one morning. The noise of jackhammers and the trucks was very loud. Theo could not concentrate on his favorite game show. He turned off the television and spent the rest of the morning pacing around the living room.

Theo usually helped Bea make sandwiches for lunch but could not concentrate and kept stopping as the noise continued. He finally went to the front door and started to go out. He appeared very angry, and Bea was afraid he would run in front of the trucks or, at the very least, start shouting at the workers. She stepped in front of him and told him to stop. He then transferred his anger to her, told her "No," and pushed her against the doorjamb. He ran out the door, waved his arms, and told the workers they had to stop. A next-door neighbor, who often helped Bea out and knew Theo had dementia, finally approached Theo calmly and got him to go back inside with him.

After the incident Bea assessed what she had done wrong. She realized that the loud noises had made Theo upset and that, because she had stepped in front of him, he had transferred his anger to her. She also realized that the neighbor stepping in when she was not there was what is called a "change of face." It is when a calm person not associated with the original problem is able to step in and distract an angry person with dementia. They had discussed it in a support group.

The next day the work continued. Bea put on soft music to mask the noise a little and led Theo to the television in the bedroom—at the back of the house—to watch his show. When she saw him getting a little angry and heading for the front door, she called him back softly. She did not mention the noise but told him she needed his help with something in the backyard (away from the noise). She gave him the hose to water the garden because he always enjoyed this. She did not hover over him asking if he was all right; had she done so, she might have become part of the problem again. She stayed inside watching him through the window, and she could tell when he became more relaxed. When he was calm, she went out, did not mention the incident, and thanked him for watering. They went for a drive and had lunch out to avoid the noise for the rest of the afternoon. When they got back, Bea again turned on soft music. Fortunately, the roadwork was completed by the end of that day, and they did not have to cope with the noise again.

Caregivers: Try not to worry too much. You may never face a catastrophic reaction with your partner, but it is best to be prepared!

4 Safety for You and Your Family Member with Dementia

Goal: This chapter will help you protect yourself and your partner in three different ways. It will tell you how to use good body mechanics when assisting your partner to move about; protect both of you from infection through the use of good infection-control techniques; and make your home environment safe.

Use Good Body Mechanics

Using good body mechanics means using your body in the correct and safe way for tasks such as lifting or moving objects or helping someone up or down to a chair or bed. Good posture, balance, and the use of your largest and strongest muscles are very important. We must all use good body mechanics to protect our backs and other muscles all the time and certainly in caregiving.

Body mechanics are ways the parts of your body work together when you move. Good body mechanics require good body alignment, using your center of gravity, and having a base of support. It will save you energy, and it will prevent injury when you push, pull, or lift objects or assist your partner.

s. Smith needed to get her husband, Henry, ready to go to the day
e center at 9:00 A.M. At 7:45 she woke him up to get dressed. She
l him that he must get up. Ten minutes later she went back to the
room, and he was still lying in bed.

enry did not understand her directions, did not remember them,
did not have the organization of movement skill necessary to sit
bed. Mrs. Smith became stressed and frustrated. She knew she
help him sit up. She then:

d to relax and took time to think through how to get her hus-
d up from bed.
ssed the room for safety, adjusting the position of the chair
e he would sit.
herself slow down, realizing that she hadn't allowed enough
she resigned herself to arriving at the center late.
sure she communicated well with Henry; she told him what
s doing and what she needed him to do as she helped him,
step (see chap. 3 for information on good interaction tech-

Dangling is an odd term, but it is important when as-
r partner to get up safely, and it is important for you
refers to sitting at the side of the bed for one to three
gain balance and adjust to an upright position before
It is a good practice for all of us as we grow older.

 one from one position and place to another is called
In addition to the use of good body mechanics, it
ep in mind several basic points when transferring:

her has a weak side due to injury or illness, plan
that the stronger side is moved first.
ay be safer to use a gait/transfer belt (a wide can-

Good Posture

Lifting and moving things are common tasks, and there are correct ways to do them. When you are performing these tasks, use good posture. You should have your:

- head erect
- shoulders back
- buttocks pulled in
- chest high
- stomach muscles tight
- back straight (as you begin to lift)

Good Body Alignment

Good alignment—having your body parts in the proper relationship to one another—is the heart of good posture and is essential to good body mechanics. Remember when your mother used to say, "Sit up straight"? When you did, your body was aligned well. When your body is in good alignment, several good things happen:

- You have more lung capacity and can breathe more easily.
- Blood circulates better, food digests easily, and your kidneys function more efficiently.
- Your body is in balance and is better protected from muscle strain and injury.
- You avoid complications from immobility, such as contractures and muscle atrophy.

For your body to be in good alignment, you need to:

- Keep a wide base of support. This will keep you more stable while you move or lift your partner. Your feet should be twelve inches, or hip width, apart. Your feet are your foundation.

- Have a stable center of gravity. Your center of gravity is the point where the most weight is concentrated in your body. When you are standing, your weight is centered in your pelvis. When you lift or move something, you must bend your knees so that your center of gravity is lower, giving you more stability. Bend your back as little as possible in the movement. This protects you from injury and falls.

Use good body mechanics whenever you lift or move something because even small lifting tasks can cause injury. Be sure to use them when:

- cleaning a floor
- carrying trash or the trash can
- picking up and/or carrying luggage
- putting things in the closet
- helping your partner adjust him- or herself
- taking off your partner's shoes or pants when he or she is in a chair or bed
- helping your partner into or out of the bathtub or shower

Transferring, Positioning, Lifting, Ambulation, and Use of Assistive Devices

Ensuring your and your partner's safety when you are transferring, positioning, lifting, and ambulating him or her depends on the use of good body mechanics. There are several other important safety guidelines.

Think ahead. You must assess the load and the stress on your body that a task will cause. As a caregiver, you may be taking on some additional household chores that you are not used to doing. When you are tired or stressed, you tend to forget to "think before you act." You may pick up something or move something

without paying any attention. When you are
is even more important to assess whether or
task safely.

Walk through the task mentally first. You
by using good body mechanics and other r
positioning or transferring, you are physic

If you have any doubt about it, ask a n
ber to help. If any aspect of caring for y
uous for you, you may need to consider
iest tasks. If you continue to do it alone
and then you and your partner will bo
the risk.

Assess the environment for safety. (
hand safely in the existing envi
through which you must move)?
Is the floor wet? Is the telephone

Communicate with your partne
decide exactly what you are g
bal cues to use before starting.
municate verbally, you shoul
Just because the person can
mean he or she does not un
you are about to do verball
ual cues).

Allow extra time when
one who has dementia
of success is for your r
has always done, the
one up for failure. Th
function the way he
same amount of tir

vas belt that fits around the waist of the one you are assisting
to transfer or walk).

- Be sure the furniture involved (bed and chair or wheelchair,
for example) will not move or tip. Make sure a wheelchair is
locked.
- Give yourself plenty of room. Check your environment (for
example, see if the wastebasket, towel rack, chair, or footstool
in the bathroom are out of your way or are positioned where
you need them).

Positioning

Positioning is moving a person into a more comfortable or beneficial body position. Too much pressure on one area for too long
can cause a decrease in circulation.

Correct positioning helps a person obtain good body alignment and promotes well-being and comfort.

Changing positions frequently prevents muscle stiffness and
skin breakdown. Pressure sores from skin breakdown are very
dangerous because they can become very difficult to heal.

To position someone correctly, remember to use good body
mechanics. You may need:

- pillows to provide support
- positioning devices (such as a back rest, a wheelchair positioning cushion, or other items to help with good body alignment and prevent complications from incorrect positioning)

Figure 4-1 shows the proper positioning for someone lying
in bed.

Lifting

When lifting your partner, you will need to use good body mechanics. Remember to:

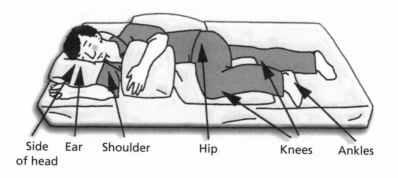

Side of head   Ear   Shoulder   Hip   Knees   Ankles

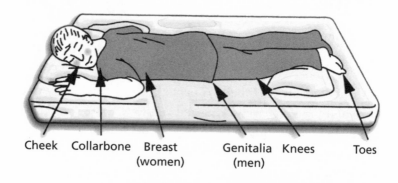

Cheek   Collarbone   Breast (women)   Genitalia (men)   Knees   Toes

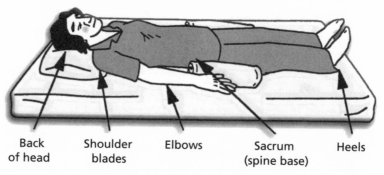

Back of head   Shoulder blades   Elbows   Sacrum (spine base)   Heels

Fig. 4-1. Proper positioning for lying in bed.

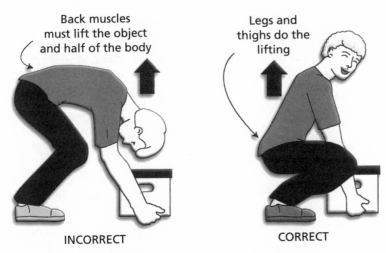

Fig. 4-2. Incorrect and correct lifting technique.

- assess your load
- check your base of support
- face what you are lifting
- bend your knees
- contract your stomach muscles as you begin the lift

Figure 4-2 shows correct and incorrect lifting techniques.

Ambulation

A person's ability to walk is called "ambulation." It is important that we all walk regularly. Even a few times around the block each week with your partner can make a difference in oxygen intake, decreased stress, increased lung expansion, and strengthened muscles. It can also be a time to become closer to your loved one as you are outside enjoying life together.

You need to make walking inside and out safe for your partner. You must be a scout, looking out for dangers ahead. Your partner's shoes should be skid resistant and must fit well. Shoestrings must be tied. The area in which you are walking must be free of clutter and anything your partner could trip over. During walks outside, watch for sidewalk cracks, uneven edges, branches, stones, and sudden changes in level. Hold your partner's arm to steady him or her and walk more slowly in areas that appear uneven. Make sure your partner uses that walker or cane if he or she has one!

Assistive Devices

If your loved one uses a cane or walker, you will need to know the correct way to use these assistive devices to prevent falls or muscle strain. Ask your physician first and then, when you purchase a device, make sure the salesperson provides a demonstration *and* written instructions with a diagram. (Important: You may be able to be reimbursed for the purchase of this equipment through Medicare or your health insurance if you have a doctor's prescription.)

Use Standard Precautions for Infection Control

Safety in the home includes removing risks of infection. Standard precautions are effective methods of infection control used by medical professionals. You must treat all body fluids as if they are infectious. Even though they did not necessarily say it in these terms, this is why your parents taught you to wash your hands after you use the bathroom.

Hand Washing

The easiest and most important way to fight the spread of infection is to wash your hands properly. Hand washing reduces the spread of disease and provides significant benefit with little or no effort or cost. Clean hands can't prevent colds because many viruses are transmitted through the air when an infected person coughs or sneezes; however, many viruses can cling to skin or inanimate surfaces such as doorknobs and railings.

The quick-and-easy hand washing done by most of us does not remove the risk of infection. It is important not to touch any dirty utensils or parts of the bathroom that are not clean during and after hand washing. This includes the sink, faucets, soap dish or container, and wastebasket. Here is a list of hand washing steps using standard precautions:

1. Turn on warm, running water. Do not touch the inside of the sink as you wash.
2. Wet your hands and wrists thoroughly under the running water. Keep your hands lower than your elbows to keep dirty water from running back down to hands.
3. Use enough soap to work up a good lather.
4. Rub your hands together and your fingers between one another.
5. Drag your nails over the palms of your hand to clean them. Rub for fifteen to twenty seconds (or the time it takes you to sing the "Happy Birthday" song).
6. Rinse your hands well. Keep them pointed downward.
7. Dry your hands with a clean paper towel, not cloth. Use the same paper towel to turn off the faucet. Toss it in the wastebasket.

When should you wash your hands?

- before and after any type of personal care (yours or your partner's)
- before and after meals
- before handling food
- before taking or giving medicine
- after sneezing or coughing
- after using the bathroom

Clean/Dirty Areas

If you have a bout with the flu, cold, or other infectious disease in your home, establish "clean/dirty areas." You may already do this without thinking. It simply means having a separate area for all laundry (clothes, bedclothes, towels) contaminated with infection. Keep dirty laundry that is not infectious elsewhere. Be sure to wash the two types separately as well.

Make Your Environment Safer

Falls: A Danger in the Home for All of Us

Some 60 percent of all falls occur in the home. About one-quarter of them are a result of hazards that can usually be avoided with careful planning and minor environmental changes.

Falls are a common reason for early admission to long-term care for all aging adults. The risk is greater for patients with dementia because the disease causes an inability to understand and correctly move about in the environment. Medications can cause confusion, dizziness, and loss of balance, resulting in falls. When this happens to a person with dementia, if the environment is unsafe as well, it is a "fall waiting to happen."

Look at all medications. Watch for prescription overdose and potentially dangerous combinations, including over-the-counter medications, herbal remedies, and alcohol.

Be aware of your own risk for falling. Fatigue or stress can damage your health and safety and can impair your ability to provide safe care. Age-related conditions, such as decreased vision, can affect all of us. Therefore, we all need to be aware of environmental adaptations to maximize safety.

The most risky areas of a home are the living room, bedroom, and hallway floors and the stairways. Bathrooms and the kitchen are the two most dangerous rooms.

Box 4-1. Common Falling Hazards

Loose throw rugs, runners, and mats

Curled carpet edges

Electrical cords

Small objects in pathways

Uncarpeted, slippery floors

No night lights and poor lighting

Lack of a sturdy handrail

Steps in need of repair

Use of inappropriate footwear

Uneven steps

No grab bars in the tub or shower

Lack of nonskid mats or strips

Toilets too low or wobbly

Low footstools

Unstable step stools

Glare from windows

Poorly lit stairways

Most falls in the home result from hazards such as those listed in box 4-1. There are many other types of hazards in our homes which are safe for us but not for a person with dementia. These include stoves, microwaves, kitchen utensils, and shop tools. Examine your home carefully and relocate or lock up any potential hazards.

All of us need to be aware of fall hazards in our homes and at work and reduce the risks. Remember, outdoor areas can be hazardous as well.

The Fall Risk Is Greater for Your Partner

In addition to the changes of normal aging, the person with dementia loses the functions that enable all of us to walk, sit, dress, eat, and use the bathroom by ourselves (see the PALMER symptoms in chap. 1). These losses combined with the normal changes of aging make the environment very unsafe for a person with dementia. The problems a person has with decreased judgment, perception, organization of movement, ability to process information, and reacting appropriately often result in falls. Your partner can't protect him- or herself; you must protect him or her.

What You Can Do to Prevent Falls

Remember, even if your partner has no problems with the environment now, it does not mean he or she will be fine later. Make adaptations now to avoid emergency changes later. There are many things you can examine and perhaps change in your home to prevent falls.

Lighting. As we get older, we need lighting two to three times stronger for us to see well. Lighting must be uniform and minimize shadows and glare. Older eyes cannot adjust quickly to lighting changes. Therefore, we all should have increased lighting levels and rails on stairs to keep us from falling. Your partner will have even more trouble due to perceptual problems. Sudden lighting changes can cause your partner to fall or to refuse to move on.

Color contrast and/or texture. A person with dementia may misinterpret a change in carpet color or texture or a change in floor finish as a change in elevation. To prevent falls, it is helpful to provide uniform floor colors between areas your partner uses most frequently. If your partner shuffles or has *hypertonia* with an unsteady gait, thresholds and floor level changes can be dangerous fall hazards.

Obstructions and changes in level. Persons with dementia have trouble with spatial perception— judging distances, heights, and changes in level. The person may not be aware of what is around him or her. (Remember, awareness is the basis for memory; see PALMER symptoms, chap. 1.) The person may not see obstacles in the path or may misjudge the distance. For example:

- The person may misjudge the distance to a chair or its height when sitting and may fall. (To help, furniture should contrast in color with the floor.)

  The person may misjudge and fall on steps without color contrast or with poor lighting. (Add good lighting and some type of a color contrast strip to edges.)
- The person may be frightened to walk on a shiny waxed floor that he or she perceives as wet or icy. (Reduce or eliminate wax.)

Seating. Most people with dementia eventually need some help getting in and out of chairs. Make sure seats are not too deep or too high. Chair arms provide leverage and will help a person remain steady. Never use chairs with wheels. Dementia can eventually affect balance. People with moderate or severe dementia may lean to one side. Even sitting upright in a chair or on a toilet can pose a danger of falling. You need non-tip chairs with good backs and sides. You may need belts on raised toilet seats to make your partner secure.

Wandering, Pacing, and Falls

People with dementia frequently wander or pace. It is difficult to understand how someone who has lived in the same home for twenty-five years can now trip over a coffee table that has always been in that same spot, yet, because of problems with awareness and perception, the person could trip and fall. There are things you can do to reduce your partner's risk of falling:

- Make sure pathways are free of obstacles. Secure extension cords, remove loose rugs, and move intruding furniture.
- Watch for exhaustion. When your partner is tired, he or she may lose balance more easily and fall. You may need to guide your partner to a chair and sit with him or her to encourage the person to rest.

- If your partner paces or wanders at night, make sure the lighting is adequate. Eliminate shadows. Falls are more common at night.

The Role of Medications in Falls

Medications can have side effects ranging from the need to use the bathroom more frequently (usually at night) to loss of balance and dizziness. These can be normal side effects (talk to your physician and pharmacist to clarify) or side effects from over-medication, combining medications improperly, or combining medications with alcohol. Keep in mind that medications include prescriptions, over-the-counter medications, and herbal medications. Side effects of improper combinations and overmedication can cause serious falls.

How to Prevent Other Types of Accidents in the Home

There are many other types of hazards you need to remove when your partner has dementia (see box 4-2 for more examples). You need to:

- Secure the stove by removing burners or putting an on/off switch inside a cabinet (turns off electricity to an electric stove).
- Put "child-proof" latches on cabinets containing dangerous products or, if possible, put the products in a part of the house to which your partner does not have access (don't forget to safety-proof the garage and/or shop area too).
- Lock doors to unsafe areas.
- Install alarms on doors, windows, and outdoor gates if your partner wanders.
- Reduce faucet hot water temperature.
- Put plastic plugs in unused outlets.

Box 4-2. How Safe Is Your Home?

	Yes	No	Corrected
Are all runners and carpets slip resistant?	❑	❑	❑
Are throw rugs removed?	❑	❑	❑
Is carpeting free from buckling?	❑	❑	❑
Are your floors free from wax so they are not slippery?	❑	❑	❑
Do you keep clutter off the floor?	❑	❑	❑
Do you remember to put dining room or kitchen chairs back in place so they will not be tripping hazards?	❑	❑	❑
Have you removed low footstools that could cause tripping?	❑	❑	❑
Have you removed glass tables and those with sharp corners?	❑	❑	❑
Have you used contrasting colors to make things like stairs, doorways, and tables more visible to your partner? (Don't forget the bathroom!)	❑	❑	❑
Do all indoor or outdoor steps provide secure footing?	❑	❑	❑
Are handrails in place by all steps, and are they secure?	❑	❑	❑
Do you have a safe step stool so you don't have to climb on a box or furniture to do a job?	❑	❑	❑

(continued)

Box 4-2. How Safe Is Your Home? *(continued)*

	Yes	No	Corrected
Is furniture off of electrical cords, to avoid causing damage resulting in a shock or fire hazard?	❑	❑	❑
Are electrical cords safely secured, not with nails or staples? Are they free of fraying and cracks?	❑	❑	❑
Are extension cords carrying no more than the manufacturer's recommended electrical load?	❑	❑	❑
Are switches and electrical outlets safe? (They should not feel warm to the touch.)	❑	❑	❑
Are light bulbs the proper size (wattage) for the fixtures?	❑	❑	❑
Do you have more than one phone, strategically placed, so you can get to a phone easily in an emergency?	❑	❑	❑
Are all emergency numbers posted near a telephone (nearest neighbor, next of kin, poison control, police, fire, doctor, 911)?	❑	❑	❑
Is there a smoke detector on each floor of your home?	❑	❑	❑
Are the smoke detectors in working order?	❑	❑	❑

	Yes	No	Corrected
Are heaters/stoves out of reach of your partner? Are they kept away from anything flammable (towels, clothing, drapes, etc.)? Mount heaters high on walls so they are out of reach.	❑	❑	❑
Do you have a professional check your furnace before you use it each year?	❑	❑	❑
Do you know how to shut off main electrical and gas lines to the house and the valves on your furnace, stove, water heater, and such? Do you know how to shut off water to your house and to individual sinks and tubs?	❑	❑	❑
Do you have an evacuation route in your house in case of fire?	❑	❑	❑
Do you have earthquake and other emergency supplies? Are they easily accessible?	❑	❑	❑
Are you careful to keep clothing (such as loose sleeves) and dish towels away from the hot stove when you cook?	❑	❑	❑
Can your stove be adapted so your AD partner cannot turn it on?	❑	❑	❑
Have you removed any countertop appliances that could cause injury?	❑	❑	❑
Is medication out of reach of an AD patient and/or children?	❑	❑	❑
Do you keep all medication in the original container?	❑	❑	❑

(continued)

Box 4-2. How Safe Is Your Home? (continued)

	Yes	No	Corrected
Do you dispose of outdated medication correctly, not in the trash?	❑	❑	❑
Have you checked the medicine cabinet and removed any potential hazards?	❑	❑	❑
Have you checked in the garage and under sinks for unsafe products that could be accessible to your partner?	❑	❑	❑
Are matches locked up?	❑	❑	❑
Are your plants inside and outside of your house nonpoisonous?	❑	❑	❑
Does your bathtub or shower have a nonskid mat?	❑	❑	❑
Do you have grab bars near your bathtub and toilet?	❑	❑	❑
Have the grab bars been installed so they are secure?	❑	❑	❑
Have you installed adjustable blinds inside and outdoor umbrellas or awnings to shield your partner's eyes from the glare of the sun?	❑	❑	❑
Are hallways and rooms well lit?	❑	❑	❑
Can you turn on lights without first walking through a dark area?	❑	❑	❑
Do you have a nightlight in the bathroom and hallway?	❑	❑	❑

	Yes	No	Corrected
Do you use electric blanket and heating pads safely?	❑	❑	❑
Is your hot water heater set no higher than 120 degrees?	❑	❑	❑
Have locks been removed from your bathroom doors?	❑	❑	❑
Are there alarms on all exterior doors and windows?	❑	❑	❑
If your car has power window controls on the passenger side, are they disabled?	❑	❑	❑
Has your car's passenger side door lock been adapted so the passenger cannot unlock it?	❑	❑	❑

It's *not* too difficult to create a safe environment for your family member.

Olivia invited her sister Yvette, who has dementia, to come and live with her. Once Yvette adjusted to the new situation, it appeared that Olivia's dining room was going to be one of her favorite places. She liked to sit at one side of the dining room table and look out the large window across the room. She usually fiddled with the small objects Olivia had on display on the buffet or rummaged in the buffet to look for things to hold and move about. Olivia decided it was better to redo the dining room than constantly have to steer her sister to other areas of the house or worry about her favorite dishes and mementoes.

Olivia moved dishes and other valuable dining room objects to the kitchen and moved unbreakable plastic containers and inexpensive utensils (nothing sharp!) from the kitchen to the dining room. She also added other things Yvette liked to the buffet drawers and shelves: yarn, fabric squares, colorful magazines, postcards, costume jewelry. She changed the items frequently so Yvette had new things to examine. In addition, she added plastic gliders—*not wheels*—to the bottom of the chairs to make them move more easily on the rug. She put double-sided tape on the bottom edges of the rug to ensure that Yvette wouldn't trip on it. She put child-proof plugs in unused outlets and taped up (shortened) the cord on the one lamp so that Yvette wouldn't trip over it. She also increased the wattage of the overhead light so there would be fewer shadows in the evening.

5 The Necessities of Daily Life
Getting Things Done with, Not Just for, Your Loved One

Goal: This chapter will help you and your partner accomplish the basic *Activities of Daily Living* (ADLs), with the least possible stress. ADLs include eating, bathing, grooming, transferring, walking (or getting about with an assistive device), toileting, continence care, and dressing. (Transferring and walking were discussed in chap. 4.)

The chapter will help you:

- understand what excess disability is and how to avoid it
- understand good nutrition for you and your partner and the unique nutritional and eating concerns for your partner with dementia
- understand bathing and grooming problems that your partner may have and how to avoid battles while dealing with them
- deal with toileting and continence care effectively as the disease progresses
- enable your partner to continue to dress him- or herself for as long as possible

Understanding Excess Disability and How to Avoid It

Excess disability is incapacity a person displays that is greater than his or her true disability. Excess disability happens because, for one reason or another, a person with dementia is not doing all the things that he or she is still able to do.

Think about your own caregiving situation. Could your partner do more than he or she is currently doing by him- or herself? Could your partner perform a task more easily if you allowed more time? Do you do things for your partner just because it seems easier that way? Do you help your partner because he or she seems to be having more difficulty than previously? Could your partner do more if you gave him or her simple, one-step instructions?

Remember that if you use all those good interaction techniques discussed in chapter 3, you will probably have better luck keeping your partner involved in his or her own ADLs. Those techniques are important to use all the time.

Your definition of success for your partner must change as the dementia changes him or her. If you do not assess your partner regularly and adapt the amount of help you're providing accordingly, you may either not help enough or help too much. Either way, you will create an excess disability. If you don't help enough, the person may refuse to finish the task, may quit before it is done, or may do it incorrectly. If you help too much, the task will get done, but the person will not use his or her remaining skills and may decline more rapidly as a result.

Always remember: If a person with dementia does not use skills, he or she will lose them. It is truly "use it or lose it" for an Alzheimer patient.

Betty is caring for her mother, Salina. Betty is the sole support for both of them and must work full-time. Salina attends an Alzheimer day care program five days a week, from 9:00 A.M. to 5:00 P.M.

Once Salina is up, she dresses and eats breakfast independently while Betty gets dressed herself—at least Betty thinks she does! This morning Betty notices that her mother is not eating breakfast. She encourages her mother to eat, reminding her that they have to leave soon. Ten minutes later Betty checks on her again, and she has eaten only a few bites. Betty is very concerned that she will be late for work and sits down and starts feeding her mother. Is Betty creating an excess disability for her mother?

Goal: For Betty's mother to keep functioning as well as possible, given her level of impairment due to AD

Problems Meeting the Goal

- Betty is expecting her mother to function as she always has and in the same amount of time.
- Betty is not aware that her mother has declined because she has not assessed her skills regularly.
- Betty has not figured out how to adapt tasks for her mother without taking over completely.

She will not create an excess disability by feeding her mother occasionally, but, if she takes over most or all of the time, she *will* create an excess disability.

Approaches to Try

- Betty should accept that her mother is declining due to dementia. She should realize that she is not failing as a caregiver because her mother can no longer do all she used to.
- Betty should assess her mother's skills regularly—all her ADLs, not just eating.
- Betty should think through how to help without doing too much. She must allow more time and guide her mother step by step. She should do as little as possible but help when needed.

Nutrition and Eating

Many ailments common to older adults are due to poor nutrition—inadequate intake of essential nutrients, dietary fiber, and water. As you care for your partner with AD, you must take care of yourself as well. You cannot provide good care if you have poor health due to poor nutrition.

A balanced diet is not difficult to carry out. Check with your physician about any additional dietary restrictions you or your partner should follow. A balanced diet should include:

- fish, legumes (beans), nuts, or dairy products as a substitute for meat as often as possible
- lots of vegetables and fruit
- whole grain breads and pasta (fiber)
- six to eight glasses of water or other fluid every day
- sparing amounts of red meat (lean only), foods high in saturated fat, sugar, and salty foods

A balanced diet will help you and your partner:

- maintain muscle and skin tissue
- maintain energy level
- maintain a healthy immune system
- cope with stress
- prevent pressure sores

Poor nutrition is common in persons with dementia because they have difficulty eating and may not eat balanced meals as a result. Even though eating is a habitual skill, something we have done all of our lives, it takes concentration and attention. It can be complicated when there are different items to eat in front of us and different types of utensils to use. In addition, different things we eat feel differently in the mouth and must be chewed and swallowed differently. Choking problems are all too common in patients with dementia. Never leave your partner alone when he or she is eating.

You may want to pat yourself on the back just because you manage to get your partner to eat something, but it is very important that the person eat a balanced diet.

Goals

- continued enjoyment of meals
- safe eating: avoidance of choking
- weight maintenance
- adequate calorie/nutrients, especially protein
- vitamin/mineral supplementation
- adequate water (the ability to store water declines with age)
- good oral hygiene
- avoidance of urinary tract infections, and constipation/diarrhea

Problems Meeting Goals

- You may be forcing food, scolding if the person does not eat, pressuring the person to eat, or rushing the person.
- You may not be paying enough attention to chewing and swallowing, which can cause choking.
- Your partner may be finding the environment noisy or confusing.
- Meal times may be inconsistent.
- Your partner may be facing too many choices.
- Your partner's glasses, dentures, or hearing aids might not be in place or not fitted properly.
- Your partner may be unable to understand how to use utensils.
- Your partner may be unable to recognize food as food or to recognize the type of food.
- The person might be "pocketing" food (keeping it in a corner of the mouth instead of swallowing).

- The person may be having trouble transitioning from chewing to swallowing because these require two separate facial movements.

Approaches to Try

Reminder: Meals should be pleasant, attractive, flavorful, and safe. Do not adapt or assist with meals more than is needed. Even mildly impaired patients, however, should probably not eat alone. They usually do not need adapted food or assistance but monitor them for any signs of a decline in functioning.

- Plan meals and make shopping lists. Prepare food ahead of time and freeze some of it. This will help you find the time for nutritious meals, reduce your stress, and keep you from buying fast food (at least most of the time!).
- Simplify meals, as needed.
- Make food colorful and well flavored.
- If your partner seems confused about what is on the plate, tell the person what he or she is eating and then remind him or her throughout the meal. Also remind the person to chew slowly.
- If the person is confused by too many items, present them one at a time.
- If the person eats poorly, try bigger breakfasts. Patients are usually hungrier in the morning.
- Provide beverages in a mug because it is easier to handle than a glass.
- Make sure food and beverages are not too hot because the person may be unable to determine temperature.
- For moderately impaired patients try soft, thick foods, which are less likely to cause choking. Combining liquids and solids, such as ready-to-eat cereal and cold milk, makes it difficult for the person to know whether to chew or swallow. Offer a drink

after every few bites to aid swallowing, but not after every bite because it is difficult to switch between the two activities.

- Break down eating into simple steps. Wait for the person to respond to an instruction before going on to the next one. For example, say, "Pick up the spoon," and then wait until he or she does so before proceeding with the next step: "Open your mouth." Keep telling the person to chew and when to swallow. If he or she cannot follow verbal cues, use touch and guide the person's hand (this is called "patterning").

- If your partner refuses to eat and you have tried everything you can think of, try the liquid nutritional supplements. They taste good and provide a person with all the needed daily nutrients.

Bathing

Bathing and shampooing the hair can be real challenges as dementia progresses. Your partner may have trouble processing all the stimuli. There are many things happening at once: the change in room temperature, the sound of water, getting undressed, feeling uncomfortable undressed, getting wet.

Try to imagine how doing these tasks feels to your partner. Put yourself in the other person's shoes. The key is simplifying the tasks, instructing one step at a time, and demonstrating as needed. Also, do the tasks really need to be done? If it is a really difficult task, pick your battles!

Remember how important a sense of security and self-esteem are for your partner (see chap. 3). Even if your partner is severely impaired, he or she needs to feel secure and valued as a person. Try to keep a consistent schedule for bathing. Do not expect the person to bathe when tired or anxious. The person's traditional bathing time is usually best. Give the person as much control as you can over the bathing process. It is very important that he or she maintain a sense of dignity and as much privacy as possible.

Mrs. Ayers now needs assistance with bathing and is embarrassed and depressed about needing the help. She has always been a somewhat private person. Now she feels as if she is fine one day and can do nothing right the next. She is embarrassed that her husband has to help her get undressed and take a bath.

Think about it. How would you feel? Mr. Ayers helped his wife by saying: "I know this is very uncomfortable for you. But I also know you would do the same for me. There are just times in our lives that we need help from each other."

Goals

Note: Mildly impaired patients may provide most of their own care.

- Cleanse the face, hands, underarms, and perineum (genital area) daily. If the patient is incontinent, cleanse the perineum every time the underwear is changed.
- Provide a bath about twice a week. Older skin is dryer and more fragile, and bathing often can be drying. If the person enjoys bathing more frequently, however, don't change the routine. (Don't "rock the boat"!)
- Provide as much independence in bathing as possible. Remember: Avoid creating excess disability!
- Provide a familiar routine, one similar to the person's previous habits. For example, if he or she always showered every night at 8:00 P.M., keep to that routine if at all possible.
- Ensure that the bathroom is safe.
- Use bath time to assess skin for any problems: bruising, cuts, infection, rashes, or swelling. Watch for pressure sores. Check fingernails and toenails. Remember: Your partner may not be able to tell you if he or she is hurt or uncomfortable.

Problems Meeting Goals

Your partner may:

- feel that bathing is scary and confusing or feel unsafe
- feel you are intruding into his or her personal space and privacy
- have poor self-esteem due to increased dependence
- not be aware that he or she needs bathing
- have physical discomfort
- refuse to bathe

Approaches to Try

- Reduce extraneous distractions: noise (run water slowly to reduce noise), glare (use lightbulbs that mimic true daylight), change in room temperature (warm up the room ahead of time), steam (use a ceiling fan).
- Speak in soothing, soft tones. Try soft music. Stay positive and cheerful.
- For safety avoid the use of oils because they can make a floor or tub slippery. Do not use floor-height space heaters, because they can burn a person and cause fires if towels or clothing are too close. Heaters should be in the ceiling or high on the wall, out of reach. Avoid loose bathroom rugs, which could cause tripping. Also, use your fan to reduce steam because clouded vision can cause accidents.
- Use a hand-held shower nozzle for bathing and shampooing. Water hitting your partner's head will run into his or her eyes and can be confusing and uncomfortable.
- If the person resists your help, try going to a beautician or barber for shampoos.
- Keep the bathing process as private as possible. Help the person wrap up in a towel while you assist him or her in undressing. You can even let the person stay wrapped in a towel or let him or her bathe in underwear if that will help. Remember to pick your battles.

- Take each task step by step. If your partner is still fairly independent, guide the choices. For example, if Tuesday is a bath day, try saying: "Today is Tuesday, your bath day. Would you like to bathe before breakfast?" If the answer is no, then respond with, "Okay, then after breakfast." It gives the person some choice in the matter. Also, arrange bathing items in the order in which your partner will need them. If your partner is more severely impaired, guide him or her through the steps of bathing. For example, you can say: "Take the washcloth. Wash under your arm."
- Have the doctor prescribe two *therapeutic* baths per week, written as a prescription for you to show to your partner.
- Let your partner eat a favorite snack, cookie, or candy while bathing to distract him or her or try giving the person something to hold (washcloth, soap), to keep him or her from grabbing you or resisting as much.
- Comment on how good the person must feel and how good he or she looks when clean.
- If resistance is very strong, try sponge baths. Help the person clean one part of the body each day, and use dry shampoo occasionally instead of a wet shampoo.
- Although routine is important, adapt your approach, method, day, and time for a bath to how the person seems to be feeling. If he or she is having a bad day, it is not a good day for a bath.
- Allow plenty of time. Think how irritated you feel when you're rushed. If your partner becomes irritated, he or she may actively resist or strike out at you.

Keep in mind that you are doing the best that you can. Don't feel guilty if your partner is not as clean as you think he or she ought to be. The person's anger with you or distress is not worth the price, unless the person's health is at risk. Remember to pick your battles. Try not to feel guilt or regret.

Grooming

Grooming tasks are generally less problematic than bathing. Brushing the hair, applying lotion, and doing nails are all easy for a patient to understand. They are pleasant, tactile (touch) activities.

Oral care (brushing the teeth) and shaving are often difficult because:

- They are more complex activities, like bathing.
- The patient cannot see what is happening (except in a mirror).
- Lots of sensations, some not pleasant, are happening at once.

Oral Care

Doing oral care is a habitual skill, even more so than bathing. The actions are so based in habit that we do not need to think about them. This works in favor of the person with dementia, but, unfortunately, oral care is complicated, so it becomes more difficult as the disease progresses. The person must try to hold water and toothpaste in his or her mouth while brushing. There is the odd sensation of the brushing action and the odd-tasting toothpaste. Then the person must try not to swallow and must rinse out his or her mouth.

Goals

- A clean, fresh mouth, clean teeth (without decay or chips), and healthy gums
- Bathroom safety

Problems Meeting Goals

Your partner may:

- feel you are invading his or her personal space
- no longer be aware of the need for clean teeth

- state that he or she has brushed when this is not true or refuse to brush (the person may not remember and may be embarrassed)
- drink the mouthwash or use shaving cream for toothpaste (safety issues)
- not be able to recognize oral pain or discomfort
- not cooperate—for example, refuse to open his or her mouth or clamp down on the brush
- have more difficulty with dentures or resist using dentures

Approaches to Try

- Guide rather than take over.
- Brush your teeth with your partner. Show him or her what you are doing face to face or in the mirror.
- Remove dangerous products from the bathroom. Make sure only the things the person needs to use are out. Put child-proof latches on the under-sink cabinet if you must store items there. Keep mouthwash locked away after use; it could make the person ill if he or she drinks it.
- If your partner will not open his or her mouth, demonstrate or start brushing his or her front teeth.
- Check dentures frequently to make sure they are in place and that they still fit properly.
- Check plates, napkins, and wastebaskets in case the person throws dentures away.
- Observe while your partner eats. If he or she winces, chews on one side only, or stops eating sooner than usual, suspect mouth pain. Examine the mouth as much as you can. The person may need to go to the dentist, as difficult as this can be.

Shaving

Again, pick your battles. This is hard if you are used to seeing your partner freshly shaved each day, but you only have so much time and/or energy to do things. Remember that you are doing an extremely difficult job. If your partner hates to shave, it is not worth his anger and your stress to keep him shaven every day. Your relationship and your health are not worth it.

Goals

To help the person:

- maintain dignity and self-esteem
- stay comfortable
- keep his or her skin in good condition

Problems Meeting Goals

Your partner may:

- refuse to shave
- be fearful of shaving (fear the sound of an electric razor or fear cutting himself)
- want to do it himself yet is not able to do it well or safely
- insist on using a straight razor

Approaches to Try

- If your partner refuses to shave, try another time.
- See if the person is comfortable with a beard.
- Try a barber.
- Dispose of any hand razors. (Perhaps it is "lost.")

Remember: Praise and compliment your partner on how fine he looks when he is done.

Toileting and Continence Care

Incontinence, the inability to control the bladder and/or bowel, happens for various reasons, but it also occurs as dementia progresses. It is usually only an occasional problem at first, but eventually it could become a chronic condition. It begins with urinary incontinence and usually progresses to bowel incontinence as well.

Toileting and continence care can be very difficult problems. They are embarrassing and uncomfortable for your partner and can distract him or her from participating in other meaningful activities.

Continence problems are time-consuming, heavy work for you. They are the primary reason for residential care or nursing home placement.

Goals

- maintaining dignity and self-esteem
- preventing urinary tract infection
- preventing constipation and/or impaction
- preventing skin breakdown
- maintaining continence and independent toileting for as long as possible

Problems Meeting Goals

Causes of incontinence may be:

- side effects of medication
- weak pelvic muscles
- infection
- a person's inability to find the bathroom
- lack of privacy
- intake of diuretics (coffee, tea, colas)
- trouble undressing, needing assistance with clothing

- a poorly lit bathroom
- a person's fear of making a mistake
- inability to recognize the sensation of needing to void (urinate or defecate)
- inability to get out of a high bed, a chair that is too deep or soft, or a chair without arms

Approaches to Try

- Observe your loved one for specific behavioral cues indicating he or she needs to void.
- Practice behavior modification (yours and your partner's). A reminder every two hours at home is a good place to start. Then modify the schedule to suit. Stop at a bathroom every two hours when out in public to avoid accidents. Remember to tell the person privately and quietly that "it's time to use the bathroom."
- Observe the person's natural toileting routine and respond to that routine.
- Reduce consumption of caffeinated beverages. Avoid alcohol. Six to eight cups of fluid daily is usually enough. (Jell-O and popsicles count as fluid.)
- Make sure the person's clothing and underwear are easy to remove. Dementia patients, as well as those with arthritis or those who have minimal muscle strength, will have trouble with buttons, hooks, and zippers. Use sweatpants with an elastic band. Many companies have affordable, attractive clothing suitable for those who are incontinent. Buck and Buck Designs is one such company (see www.buckandbuck.com or 800-458-0600). Sears stores have also started carrying them.
- Put signs with easy-to-read words and/or pictures on bathroom doors to identify them.
- Try a commode by the bed at night. Bruce Medical Supply has useful products (800-225-8446 or www.brucemedical.com); also try the Posey Company (800-44p-osey or www.posey.com).

- Remove physical obstacles to getting to the bathroom in time.
- Try to make sure the person chooses seating that he or she can get up out of easily.
- When your partner is incontinent, treat it in a matter-of-fact manner, quietly, with understanding and empathy. Do not scold the person.
- Use the words your partner uses for going to the bathroom. Do not call it "going potty" or some such term unless the person does. If the person does use a childhood term of some sort, then that is the term to use.
- Do not call disposable underwear "diapers" unless that is the only term the person seems to respond to. Patients are usually embarrassed enough that they are incontinent and do not want to be made to feel more childish.
- Have appropriate supplies and disposable underwear in each bathroom.
- Always use disposable gloves when assisting your partner. Use a slightly larger size than your regular gloves, because you need to be able to get them on and off quickly. Dispose of them and the soiled disposable underwear immediately. Put them in a disposable trash bag without touching the soiled items. Use a container with a lid. Put it out of the reach of your partner or small children. (A cabinet with a child-proof latch would be a good choice.)
- Make sure your partner is clean and dry to prevent skin irritation, sores, and skin breakdown.
- Patients with dementia can lose the ability to concentrate on pushing and the ability to push when having a bowel movement. This can result in impactions (hard-to-move waste buildup). Fiber products such as Citrucel, Fibercon, and Bene-fiber make it easier for the person to have a bowel movement. Make sure the person drinks adequate water with fiber products to avoid choking. Water also helps prevent impaction.

- Encourage a male patient to sit to urinate. He may then also have a bowel movement, and it may help avoid messy clean-up.
- Toilet paper, washcloths, and tissues can be confused with one another. If possible, leave an appropriate amount of toilet paper and remove the other items.
- If there is a wastebasket beside the toilet, the person may void into that. Put it elsewhere. Be aware that the sink or tub can be used as a urinal by a male patient too! Pull a shower curtain across the side of the tub if there is confusion.
- Many good spot-removal products are available at home repair and grocery stores. Use white vinegar to remove urine smells. Polyester pants will retain urine smells more than others.

Dressing

Dressing is usually not a huge problem early in the disease process, but it can become one as the dementia becomes more severe. Some points to remember are:

- Always allow plenty of time.
- Simplify clothing.
- Reorganize storage spaces as needed.
- Be prepared for unusual combinations and then determine if these are suitable for the day's events. Remember to pick your battles.
- Letting the person choose clothing and dress independently is more important than being dressed perfectly in most cases.
- Be sure your partner is dressed appropriately for cold, very warm, or wet weather.

If your partner has early-stage dementia, he or she probably has little trouble dressing except for using more complicated things such as ties, blouses with tiny buttons, pantyhose, and jew-

elry with clasps. As the disease progresses, the person will probably have more difficulty. Remember to assess carefully and help
as little as possible.

Goals

- to make it possible for the person to dress him- or herself for
  as long as possible
- to help the person maintain dignity and self-esteem
- to allow for the person's personal preferences as much as
  possible
- to reinforce the person's sense of comfort and safety

Problems Meeting Goals

The person may:

- not recognize body parts
- not recognize what an item of clothing is or how to put on a
  specific type of garment
- forget that he or she has already put on a specific type of clothing and put another one on also (this type of "layering" is very
  common)
- dress inappropriately for the weather (watch for dressing too
  warmly due to layering in hot weather)
- not like someone else handling his or her belongings or, if undressing, may think you are taking his or her clothes
- not accept help because he or she is uncomfortable dressing
  and undressing in front of you or is embarrassed about needing help
- refuse to dress because it looks complicated and overwhelming
- dress in clothing that doesn't match
- want to wear the same thing every day

Approaches to Try

- Allow plenty of time. Confusion, frustration, and irritability become more of a problem when you are rushing the person. Put yourself in his or her place. Dressing can be frustrating and irritating for anyone who is rushed. If the person is irritable, he or she may resist or even strike out at you.
- Be flexible. If no one else is around or it is "just family," it is okay if the person's clothes don't match. What is important is that the person dressed him- or herself.
- Let the person choose how to dress. You will have to reduce the number of choices eventually. If the person cannot choose, try saying, "Here, this will look great on you," rather than simply, "Put this on." Stay positive and try not to make instructions sound like orders.
- When helping, cue the person in short, simple steps.
- Simplify garments. Choose slacks and socks instead of a skirt and pantyhose for a woman, for example. Avoid pantyhose and knee highs that are too tight and can cut off circulation.
- Lay out clothes in the correct order for dressing: underclothes on top, then outer clothing, then socks, then shoes on the bottom. With these extra cues the person may be able to dress on his or her own. If this doesn't work, hand the person one item at a time.
- If your partner refuses to dress or undress, wait, use the short-term memory loss to your advantage, and then approach the person later.
- Remove off-season clothing from the closet.
- If your partner rummages or puts clothing in strange places, put only one or two choices in the closet or drawers at a time. Store the rest elsewhere.
- If the person has trouble hanging clothes on hangers, lower the rods or try adding one or two rods. Your partner can then fold clothes over the rods.

- Choose shoes that are easy to put on. Avoid shoes with laces but make sure shoes are secure. No clogs or open-backed shoes!
- If the person insists on wearing the same clothes daily, wash these clothes at night or have several identical outfits.
- Does the person want to wear daytime clothing to bed? As long as the clothes are not binding and harming circulation, allow it. It is okay for the person to change clothes at odd times, when he or she is in the mood, not just by a traditional schedule. Be flexible.

A few patients, women in particular, remain very conscious of dressing well. The person usually accepts assistance easily if it is needed because he or she is concerned with looking good in public more than with dressing by him- or herself.

Whatever pleases your partner and aids his or her self-esteem is of primary importance in this case—whether it be choosing clothes, dressing independently, or looking great.

Remember: Redefine your idea of success and pick your battles. If you have helped your partner to be fairly clean, dressed, toileted, and fed and the person is doing as much as possible on his or her own, you are doing an incredible job!

6 Keeping Busy and Enjoying Time Together

Goal: This chapter will provide you with ideas for keeping your partner functioning well. It will help you keep your partner content and busy with normal tasks of everyday life and will cover some activities the two of you can share and enjoy. An additional goal is to make life easier for both you and your partner.

Busy Is Better, for Your Partner and for You

Any task we do as part of daily life is an activity. Even sleeping is an activity. A *therapeutic activity* is one that benefits the person doing it.

Most AD patients can not stay physically and mentally active on their own. You, as the caregiver, must make sure that they stay active. Chapter 5 addressed how to keep your partner involved in his or her own personal care. The basic personal care tasks of daily life, called Activities of Daily Living (ADLs), are all activities (see chaps. 1 and 5).

Staying involved in his or her own care and in other therapeutic activities may help your partner in several ways. The person may:

- keep functioning at a higher level for a longer time if he or she is keeping mind and body active and using remaining skills daily (it is "use it or lose it" for patients with dementia)
- maintain greater self-esteem and interest in daily life because he or she is doing important, adult activities
- have fewer *behavior problems* simply because he or she has something to do

Even if it is an effort at first to plan activities and get them started, activities can provide you with the breaks you need. Without breaks you will feel stressed, and your health may suffer. You can get other things done when your partner is occupied.

Doing things together that you both enjoy will increase your quality of life. It may help you remain close. It will provide good memories, even though these years may be difficult. You will both benefit physically and mentally from sharing positive experiences.

Stimulation and Activities

Like the rest of us, your partner needs different types of stimulation each day to remain as healthy and alert as possible. *Stimulation* in this context means the benefit your partner gains from a specific type of activity. If the person does not have appropriate stimulation, he or she may develop excess disability. The person may decline in health and ability to function more rapidly than necessary.

Essential types of stimulation for your partner are easy to provide in a normal day. Don't feel as if you have to plan ahead for all of them. It is hard to plan a day for a patient with dementia. The person can be alert and cooperative one minute but not the next.

Study the situation: Each evening for a few days review what your partner did that day. (The assessment diary mentioned in chap. 1 can help.) Ask yourself questions such as:

- Did my partner just sit or just pace most of the day?
- Did my partner sit alone with no one to talk to most of the day?
- Did my partner do nothing to occupy the time all day?

You may see a good mix of activities or an activity pattern that needs changing.

The important thing is variety in the types of stimulation your partner receives each day. Basic daily requirements are:

- maximum involvement in one's own ADLs
- large-motor activities: things to really stretch the muscles, such as walking around, raking leaves, or exercising with you to an exercise video or to music
- *fine motor* activities: holding and moving things around with the hands and arms, such as looking at old greeting cards, folding laundry, or doing a jigsaw puzzle
- social/emotional activities: visiting with others, hugging a grandchild, stroking a pet (even an unaware, nonverbal person needs conversation and hugs)
- rest and "down time"—unfortunately, this is usually the easiest type of activity to do; if your partner rests too much during the day, however, he or she may not sleep at night

Strictly alternating types of activities is not as important as providing different types of activities throughout the course of the day. Try to vary or alternate as follows:

- active (moving around) and passive (without much movement) activities: for example, watching "I Love Lucy" (passive) followed by a walk outside (active); or doing a jigsaw puzzle (generally passive) then getting up to feed the dog (active)
- hard (cognitively demanding) and easy (relaxing, not demanding): for example, helping to make a cake (hard) followed

by getting up to watch children play outside (easy, relaxing); or listening to music (easy, relaxing) followed by drying dishes (hard)

Remember that what is hard and easy for your partner will change with time. As the disease becomes more severe, what was once easy may become difficult. As problems with organization of movement (basic PALMER symptoms; see chap. 1) become more severe, staying active may be more difficult. Don't eliminate types of stimulation, just modify them. For example, if the person begins having more difficulty organizing his or her movements, suggest a walk on the patio, not around the block.

Keeping an AD patient busy is hard work. You are doing a good job just keeping the person healthy and safe.

If you are frail or ill or unable to cope with your partner for some other reason, consider other options. Adult day care, friends or relatives, and a home companion or home health aide are alternatives to consider for help with your partner's activity needs and care. No one expects you to endanger your own health while providing appropriate care to your partner.

Adapt Normal Activities of Daily Life for Your Partner

In addition to the ADLs there are other tasks we all do each day. These are more varied in the way we do them and more complex. They are called *Instrumental Activities of Daily Living* (IADLs). They include:

- housekeeping; work in the shop, garage, and outdoor areas (if applicable)
- doing laundry
- food preparation
- shopping

- using the telephone
- managing money
- using transportation: car, taxis, public transportation, and other types
- taking medication

Some IADLs work better than others as activities for a person with dementia. Housekeeping, doing laundry, and preparing food almost always work when adapted as activities. Activities that work for many patients, but cause anxiety or an obsession with the task in others, are shopping, using the telephone, and riding in the car. Taking medication cannot, of course, be adapted as an activity.

These activities work well because they are adult. Your partner will remember them from the past and know they are important household tasks. Even severely impaired patients often seem to remember doing IADLs and their importance. There are clear benefits for your partner to doing them:

- The person feels pride of accomplishment when finished.
- You have the supplies on hand.
- They are often things you must do anyway.

Be sure to allow plenty of time and simplify the task. Many of these tasks can be adapted and simplified to one or two steps. Because they are simple and familiar, often a patient needs only a little help.

Keep in mind that the goal of these activities is to give your partner adult, meaningful tasks and a sense of accomplishment. They are great for you because, once "engaged," your partner may do them without constant supervision from you.

Be prepared. Examine the work area and make sure it and any supplies are safe. If your partner is "helping" you, remember that it may actually slow down your work. If it is a household task, realize that you may have to do it over discretely once the person is "finished."

If the person enjoys an activity, let him or her do it repeatedly, even if it isn't needed. For example:

- If your partner likes to dry dishes, rinse unbreakable dishes deliberately so he or she can dry them.
- In the fall dump leaves back in the yard several different times. This is often successful with men, because it is adult, helpful, and "manly," and they are proud of their work when it is done.

Housekeeping

Housekeeping tasks are familiar to everyone. Try:

- Dusting. Do not use toxic chemicals. Avoid spray or aerosol bottles.
- Vacuuming, mopping, sweeping, using a duster.
- Rearranging books or unbreakable and safe office and kitchen items. (Don't care about where they actually wind up!)
- Washing windows—not on ladders. Use nontoxic vinegar and water on a rag.

Yardwork

Being outdoors can improve one's mood and lift the spirits. Outdoor tasks that work well include:

- Sweeping sidewalks and the patio.
- Weeding the yard and garden. Accommodate balance problems.
- Watering.
- Picking fruit and vegetables—not on a ladder.
- Picking and arranging flowers. Boxes of artificial flowers and unbreakable vases work well for making arrangements over and over again.

Shop and Garage Work

These activities may be especially enjoyable for male partners, who may enjoy:

- Rearranging items such as nuts and bolts, screws, and other shop items. Make sure your partner will not swallow small items. Lock up any dangerous tools or chemicals.
- Sanding wooden blocks or other simple shapes such as cutting boards. Mildly impaired patients may be able to do more complex woodwork.
- Sweeping the shop and garage.

Doing Laundry

Handling clean clothes that are warm and smell good can be a very soothing activity. Try:

- Sorting clothes. Be prepared for errors.
- Folding laundry.
- Putting clean laundry away, "arranging" it. Be prepared to do it again later when your partner is not around.

Food Preparation

Food preparation works well because it is familiar to everyone. Your partner may be able to help with even complex food preparation, one step at a time. Do not let the person use the oven or stove or sharp items. With your help, try having your partner:

- Prepare a set part of a meal each day. Perhaps he or she can always make the dinner salad.
- Prepare salsa or other dishes for which the person can chop to his or her heart's content. Use rounded table knives with serrated edges—you can find ones that do work for this!
- Shell peas or clean and ready other garden vegetables and fruit for meals.

- Set the table, one item at a time. For example, all the plates first (or maybe only the plates), then all the spoons, with you pointing to where they go, and so on.
- Wash, rinse, or dry safe and unbreakable dishes, pots, pans, and utensils. The person probably cannot do all three, just one task—washing, rinsing, or drying, while you do the rest. (Soapy water is often very soothing to anxious patients.)
- Arrange flowers, items on serving plates (such as small sandwiches or cookies), and other items for a special small party for a few family members or for just the two of you.

Shopping

Shopping is one of the more difficult IADLs. It may overwhelm some patients, and some may obsess about the cost involved. Simplify purchases and shorten trips. Your partner may enjoy:

- Helping to plan a shopping list.
- Cutting out coupons. A great activity—outline cutting marks in dark ink, so the person knows where to cut (it is okay if your partner cuts out more than you need!).
- Taking items off store shelves and putting them in the cart.
- Helping you put items in the car and unloading them at home.
- Unwrapping purchases at home and putting away groceries.
- Shopping for a specific item, such as a birthday or Christmas gift. Choose a general type of gift together ahead of time, then write it on the shopping list for your partner's reference.

Using the Telephone

The phone becomes an obsession with some patients. If this is the case, you may need to hide the phone or even disconnect it at times. Your partner may enjoy:

- A prearranged call to friends or relatives. Write down things the person wants to say ahead of time. Stay by your partner, preferably participating on a second phone, to offer prompts as needed.

- Having family and friends call the person. You should arrange it, know the topic for conversation ahead of time, and have people call at a specific time so you can help with the conversation.

Handling Money

Money can be an obsession for some patients. They may think someone is taking it or worry that they do not have enough. Nevertheless, your partner may enjoy:

- Having a small amount in a wallet, pocket, or purse, "just in case." (Make sure to remove credit cards!)
- Paying the cashier or sales person with the exact amount. (No making change!)
- Sorting and stacking coins or putting them in the coin wrappers used by banks.

Outings by Car / Travel

If your partner loved to drive and cannot anymore, he or she may be upset when you are driving (see chap. 3), yet riding in a car is a great activity for most patients. Point out interesting things to your partner because he or she may not notice them on his or her own.

Basic car safety precautions include:

- Locking the passenger doors and windows using control options on the driver's door panel.
- Deciding whether your partner will be safer in the back or front seat.
- Always having duplicate keys in your wallet or purse and somewhere outside of the car (such as in a magnetic case).

Your partner may enjoy:

- going to a specific place to picnic and walk, perhaps a park or by the ocean.
- combining a drive with errands—you can take a new or longer way if the person loves to ride.

If you cannot get your partner in and out of the car easily, try inviting friends or other family members along to help. Or just drive. Drive through new neighborhoods or parks or by the ocean. Have a picnic in the car at a pretty spot. Go to a drive-through restaurant window and then picnic in the car.

Basic travel safety precautions include:

- checking with your physician and obtaining anti-anxiety medication to give to your partner if her or she becomes anxious and confused (have your partner try out the medication in advance to evaluate his or her reaction)
- looking for unisex, family, or single-stall restrooms so you can help your partner easily; be aware that some bathrooms have two or more exterior doors
- obtaining "handicapped" assistance on planes, in airports, on trains, and on cruise ships
- checking connections ahead of time (make sure you can get home from transfer points or your destination quickly if necessary)

If your partner is only mildly impaired, a cruise may be a good choice because you can stay in one place once you get there. Be sure to purchase trip insurance in case you must cancel or leave the trip partway through.

Involve Your Partner in the Flow of Daily Life

To help your partner use remaining memory skills, involve him or her in the flow of daily life. Unless your partner has severe dementia, try to include him or her in many ordinary, everyday activities. Being involved helps the person feel secure and part of life, encourages the use of the remaining short-term memory, and may help the person retain it longer. Choose the time of day your partner is at his or her best for special events, especially those involving children.

When you go to bed at night, you probably think of all the things you need to do the next day, and often the tasks are interrelated. For example, you may plan a salad for dinner, go buy ingredients, prepare the salad, set the table, and serve the salad for dinner. Try to integrate activities for your partner into the flow of your day. For example, Mary Stevenson involved her husband, Charles, in preparing for a family visit.

Tuesday morning the Stevensons' daughter calls to say she will bring her children to visit on Thursday afternoon, the best time of day for Mr. Stevenson, who is a moderately impaired AD patient. Mrs. Stevenson, Mary, involves Charles in the plans:

- deciding what snack to serve, buying groceries, and then fixing the snack;
- setting out some toys the children keep at their grandparents' home;
- cleaning up the living room and yard so there is more room for play and visiting.

Mary tells Charles about the visit. She tells him she needs his help to get ready. She also:

- keeps reminding him of things they need to do and about the visit;
- decides what Charles can do to help, and how to do it;
- allows lots of extra time for anything he does.

Tuesday morning Mary includes Charles in choosing a snack. She shows him pictures in the cookbook so he understands. They decide on chocolate chip cookies and make a grocery list.

Tuesday afternoon they shop. They are buying only cookie ingredients and drinks. Charles puts items in the cart, then into the car, and carries them into the house. Mary reminds him of the things they are doing and the visit. She tells him they will make cookies the next day, Wednesday.

Wednesday morning she reminds him of all the following day's events, and they make the cookies together. Wednesday afternoon they look over toys, choose some, and Charles puts them on the patio. She again reminds him of the next day's events.

Thursday morning they straighten up the living room and patio. Charles moves some things out of the way and sweeps the patio. Mary reminds him of everything they are doing to prepare for their family's visit several times.

Thursday afternoon there are more reminders from Mary and the very special time with their daughter and grandchildren.

Caution: Some patients become very nervous thinking about events in the future. They may dwell on them and talk about them over and over. If this is the case with your partner, involve him or her in getting ready but don't mention the event until the actual day or even just before it takes place.

Enjoyable Activities for Your Partner and for You

Reminiscing boxes are great and can be made for free! Collect things from your garage or attic and from friends. Put different types of objects in each box. These are "no fail" activities, with no "right" or "wrong" way to do them.

Like the IADLs, reminiscing boxes can also be used for great one- or two-step activities. Persons with dementia do single-step

- Ribbons and lace
- Artificial flowers and vases
- Seashells, perhaps with some sand in a dishpan; old sand toys (for "remembering")—Keep it adult when you talk about it. For example, do not call it "playing in the sand."
- Decorations and photos for specific holidays (each holiday in a separate box)
- Sandpaper and different types and sizes of wood pieces—Make cutting boards, wooden blocks, other household objects or toys; wax or oil completed projects.
- Game pieces such as playing cards, dominoes, Jenga, or Block Head to arrange randomly or play simple games for two or more players
- A selection of baby or children's clothing
- Matchbox cars, small plastic toy animals, or other figures
- Large wooden or other types of beads and thick string (stiffened with tape or glue at the end for threading) or long shoelaces

Good One- or Two-Step Activities
If your partner has mild or moderate dementia and you engage and then reengage him or her occasionally, it can stimulate your partner to do some activities on his or her own. Others you can enjoy doing together.

Your partner may enjoy:
- Coloring an adult-looking coloring book—Take pages out of the book. It feels more like adult artwork that way. It's usually not a good idea to call it "coloring"; perhaps call it "drawing." Pick simple pictures or enlarge sections of bigger ones on a copy machine.
- Trying other types of drawing (using pencils, watercolors, chalk, colored pens, stencils, and different types of paper)
- Looking at pictures or a book or magazine with colorful pictures— *National Geographic* is a good choice. Avoid children's books unless a child is with you or you are using them for reminiscing about

(continued)

Box 6-1. Enjoyable Activities for Your Partner and for You
(continued)

times with your children or grandchildren. Although not a one- or two-step activity, reading poems or short stories together often works, too. The sound of your voice can be very soothing even if the person does not fully understand. Many patients also like to read out loud, even if they do not grasp a lot of what they are reading.

- Stuffing envelopes for local organizations, including (in some cases) folding, gluing, and stamping each envelope separately
- Kneading yeast dough (making bread, rolls, pizza dough)
- Cracking nuts
- Winding yarn—Stretch a skein between two posts or prepare pieces no longer than ten feet to keep it from getting tangled. Have your partner wind them into a single ball. Different-colored and textured pieces add appeal and look colorful when wound.
- Throwing or rolling and catching different types of balls

Box 6-2. Simplified Versions of Adult Games

Active Games
- Horseshoes—Use heavy plastic horseshoes, not metal or very light-weight children's toys.
- Lawn darts—Use weighted, not sharp-pointed ones.
- Indoor dart games—Use plastic darts and a special dart board, not metal darts.
- Shuffleboard (available on a long plastic sheet for temporary use)—Play from one end only, letting the score be where the disk lands in the opposite triangle.

6. He continued, step by step, with only the specific supplies needed for each step set out in front of them. If Julia were more severely impaired, he might do most of the steps and have her do a single one, such as stirring the batter.

Try an activity based on a past interest. Simplify it and adapt equipment as needed.

Tom used to golf. He now enjoys putting in his backyard. He uses a standard golf club and hollow plastic balls (so they will not go too far) and hits them to large, easy-to-see targets, flags, or foam circles. (Computer mouse pads make great targets.)

What if your partner is not interested? You can try:

1. Starting the activity on your own but asking the person to sit beside you to keep you company or just to sit and watch.
2. To keep talking to keep the person there and alert.
3. If the person keeps watching, saying after awhile, "Here, help me" or "Your turn!" *Don't* say, "Would you like to help?" because this often invites a no. If the person starts to participate, quietly give him or her short, simple instructions. Don't ask "Is it okay?" or "Why did you not want to do this before?" because the person may then stop again.

Why is it hard to get your partner interested? There are many possible reasons. Your partner:

- may not be aware that you are even there, may not understand that you are suggesting something to do, or may not understand what you are suggesting. Reminder: Show the equipment and samples, let the person touch the objects. Watch the person's face to see if he or she is watching and understands.
- may not understand, just by looking at the supplies or equip-

ment, that the activity might be fun. Reminder: Start it in front of the person. He or she may then "catch on."

- may resist because you are saying, "Do you want to do this?" Doing all the things we take for granted is very scary for patients with dementia, and they may have a negative response because of that. Try saying, "I'll be there to help" or "We'll do it together. It's not so hard."

- may get tired of having someone always telling him or her what to do. (Wouldn't you?) It may help the person maintain self-esteem to say no. Ask again later or do the activity in front of the person, and he or she may join in. If the person can not see you doing it, he or she will forget about it.

Rose's husband, Ben, has always been very independent and is very negative much of the time now that he needs more help doing things due to Alzheimer disease. Rose gets him to help fix lunch or dinner by inviting him to sit at the kitchen to "just talk" while she prepares the meal. She then starts making sandwiches, for example, and "happens" to move a tomato that needs slicing in front of Ben. It is on a cutting board with a serrated knife with a rounded tip. She knows he can use it safely. She then pays no attention but starts slicing another tomato nearby. She doesn't comment at all, but Ben usually then starts to do the task while they talk. She thanks him very briefly when he is done and then slides some other task in front of him.

Why does Ben finally help? He may respond because he has exerted his right to say no and then is able to start when *he* wants to. Rose doesn't embarrass him by calling the task to his attention. He also may not have understood what she wanted him to do until he saw her begin. Observing her may have triggered his response.

Glossary

acetylcholine. A neurotransmitter that sends (transmits) signals from one nerve cell (neuron) to another. The transmittal is responsible for learning and memory. Acetylcholine is severely depleted in Alzheimer disease by an enzyme called acetylcholinesterase. Medications such as Aricept stop the acetylcholinesterase from depleting the acetylcholine.

active aging. A lifestyle of an older adult who makes a conscious effort to adapt to any deficits due to aging by keeping active physically, mentally, and socially.

Activities of Daily Living (ADLs). The most basic personal care tasks we must be able to do to live independently. They are transferring (moving from one position to another, such as getting into and out of bed, a chair, or a wheelchair), toileting and continence care (cleansing oneself after using the toilet), bathing, dressing, grooming, walking or getting about with an assistive device (wheelchair or walker, for example), and eating.

agnosia. The loss of ability to recognize familiar things by sight, sound, touch, taste, or smell.

Alzheimer disease. A disease caused by lethal structural damage to the brain including tangles and plaques, with an abnormal beta-amyloid protein present in the plaques. It is always progressive, irreversible, lethal (fatal), and can be diagnosed only by autopsy.

This disease causes dementia. It is a "type of dementia" or a "dementing illness."

ambulation. The act of walking about.

apathy. Lack of feeling and emotion, lack of response or desire to act.

aphasia. A general term for loss of language abilities due to brain damage. *Expressive aphasia* is the loss of written or spoken language ability. *Receptive aphasia* is the loss of ability to understand written or spoken language.

aspiration. The act of inhaling. Aspiration pneumonia is caused by inhaled food particles in the lungs. It is a common cause of death in persons with Alzheimer disease, due to improper chewing and swallowing of food.

assessment. An evaluation or measure. In terms of caregiving, an evaluation of a person's ability to function normally. Ongoing assessment is vital to appropriate care for those with dementia.

assisted living. A long-term care community usually regulated by the state's Department of Social Services. These facilities provide supervision, personal care, and meals for residents who do not need regular or constant medical care. They are nonmedical and tend to be larger facilities or a portion of a larger retirement community. They are designed for older persons or may be for persons with dementia specifically. Residential care and "board and care" facilities are under the same license.

autopsy. A postmortem (after death) examination performed by a pathologist (a physician who studies the nature of disease) to determine cause of death or the nature of a disease process, such as Alzheimer disease.

behavior problem. A difficult behavior in a person with dementia which is harmful, potentially harmful, or disturbing to the person or others. The basic symptoms (PALMER symptoms) are not behavior problems. Behavior problems are secondary; they occur because of these basic symptoms.

benign forgetfulness. The normal slowing of some mental powers in aging.

beta-amyloid. A type of amyloid (a fibrous body protein deposit). The gene for it is on chromosome 21. A segment of this protein is in the plaques exterior to brain cells of persons with Alzheimer disease.

caregiver. A person directly or indirectly responsible (long-distance caregiving is common now) for some, most, or all of the care of another human being.

catastrophic reaction. A sudden, uncontrolled change for the worse in a person's behavior. It is common in persons with dementia and can happen for a wide variety of reasons.

chronic condition. A disease or disorder that develops slowly and persists over a long period of time. Alzheimer disease is a chronic condition.

cognition. The process of thinking and learning. All of the PALMER symptoms (the basic symptoms of dementia) involve cognitive abilities. Alzheimer disease causes general loss of cognitive abilities (disability).

delusion. A false belief a person maintains despite provable evidence to the contrary. Delusions are common in dementia.

dementia. A global loss of intellectual functioning or cognition caused by disease or injury to the brain. Dementia is not a normal part of aging. Alzheimer disease is the most common form of dementia.

diagnosis. Identification of a disease or condition through scientific observation and assessment of symptoms using various procedures (for example, lab work, X rays, and personal history).

differential diagnosis. A complex diagnosis based on differentiating symptoms from other conditions with similar symptoms. Alzheimer disease cannot be confirmed except through an autopsy. A thorough differential diagnosis can eliminate other causes of dementia, however, with a 99 percent accuracy rate compared to autopsy results.

disease. Any deviation of normal body function or structure which can be identified by specific symptoms or other characteristic signs. The term *disease* does not mean a condition is contagious or transmittable to others.

excess disability. The disability a person displays beyond what should be present as a result of the true level of impairment.

fine motor skills. The ability to use muscles in the body in small, precise movements (for example, using fingers, wrist, hand, and arm movements to write or draw).

formulary. A listing of medications available at a pharmacy or through a health care plan and from which physicians can prescribe. Many health plans will cover only generic drugs listed in the formulary.

hallucination. A persistent sensory perception—something a person sees, hears, smells, or feels in the external world when nothing is really there.

hippocampus. A small area deep in the brain, at the base of the cerebrum, which is responsible for memory and learning. It is the first area of the brain affected in Alzheimer disease.

hospice. Medically supervised end-of-life care. Its goal is to make the person as comfortable as possible, without treatments to try to cure or prolong life. Hospice support is available to families as well. It is available in almost all residential long-term care settings and at home.

hypertonia. Increased muscle resistance to bending or stretching, causing stiffness and rigidity.

incontinence. The loss of bowel and/or bladder control due to physical problems or to an inability to perceive the body's signals correctly. It is common in moderate and severe Alzheimer disease.

Instrumental Activities of Daily Living (IADLs). Necessary tasks of daily life (shopping, preparing meals, housecleaning, doing laundry, managing money, using transportation, using the telephone, taking medication) which are not as crucial to independent living as ADLs. They also vary widely in methods of implementation (ways of doing them).

large motor skills. The ability to use muscles of the body in wide, expansive movements (for example, using the muscles of the legs and arms to dance, walk, or lift).

long-term care. Professional care provided on a regular basis for a long period of time. There are many long-term care options, including, among others, home companion and nursing care, social and adult day health care, residential and assisted living, nursing homes, and hospice services. Specialized dementia-specific care is available in all types of long-term care settings.

mild cognitive impairment (MCI). Mild damage to the brain resulting in some loss of intellectual functioning.

passive aging. Inactivity (physically, mentally, or socially) due to an inability or lack of desire to adapt well to the normal aging process.

pathology. The branch of medicine which explores or determines the nature of a disease by examining tissue and organs to determine structural and functional changes.

perception. The registration in the brain of sensory stimulation—things seen, felt or touched, heard, tasted, or smelled.

perseveration. The tendency of persons with dementia to repeat the same actions, sounds, or words over and over. It can be a severe behavioral problem, but therapeutic activities consisting of one or two simple steps use the tendency to perseverate to good advantage.

positive interaction techniques. Appropriate, positive verbal and nonverbal communication methods that work best with persons with dementia to maintain a positive emotional climate and positive working relationship.

reengage. To reorient someone to a task when he or she appears to be losing interest or to have forgotten what he or she is doing. A person with dementia requires this assistance due to the short attention span.

residential care facility. A small long-term care community (also called a "board and care") usually regulated by a state's Department of Social Services Community Care Licensing division. It is nonmedical and is not required to have nurses or a resident physician. It tends to be ten beds or fewer and a private home or intended to be homelike. Some facilities are specifically for younger residents, older residents, or those with dementia. Assisted living facilities tend to be larger but are under the same license in most states.

senility. An inappropriate, outdated term referring to the slow deterioration of mental functions during the aging process. It was used to mean forgetfulness in aging believed to be normal. Severe forgetfulness is not normal.

sensory. Of the basic senses—visual, auditory (hearing), tactile (touch or feeling), olfactory (smell), and taste. Sensory stimulation refers to actions or activities that make use of the basic senses in some way. Even persons with very severe dementia retain some use of the basic senses.

skilled nursing. A long-term care community licensed by a state's Department of Health Services. It is for those who need constant medical care and supervision. Licensed nurses, certified nurse assistants (CNAs), and a resident physician are required by licensing. There are skilled nursing facilities specifically for persons with dementia, and many have dementia care units.

step. A simple message or action complete in itself, one that does not require remembering other steps to understand and complete it. Most persons with dementia need instructions divided into individual, easy-to-understand components, or steps. For example, "pick up the book" is a one-step instruction. "Pick up the book and open it to page 5" is a two-step instruction and would be difficult for many people with dementia.

sundowning. Confusion, restlessness, lack of concentration, and irritability common in persons with dementia toward the end of the day. The cause is not known, but it happens, at least in part, because the person is "overloaded" and extremely tired by the end of a long day due to reduced cognitive functioning.

therapeutic. Beneficial or healing, designed to maximize a person's self-esteem.

therapeutic activity. An activity designed to maximize a person's everyday functioning (including but not limited to ADLs and IADLs) and feeling of well-being. It should feel purposeful to the person and should be designed to increase his or her self-esteem.

therapeutic program. A total plan of care based on assessment of a person's level of functioning. It is designed to reduce excess disability, difficult behaviors, and other secondary symptoms of dementia.

ventricles. The two central areas of the brain which contain cerebrospinal fluid.

Resources

The Alzheimer's Association provides dementia-specific referrals, support groups, volunteer respite, caregiving training, and support (phone: 800-272-3900; national Web site: www.alz.org).

The Alzheimer's Disease Education and Referral (ADEAR) Center is a service of the National Institute of Aging (NIH) and is an invaluable source of nationwide information (phone: 800-438-4380; email: adear@alzheimers.org; Web site: www.alzheimers.org).

The National Institute on Aging, Alzheimer's Disease Education and Referral (ADEAR), is a good source of information on finding reputable clinics, among other things (phone: 800-438-4300).

Perspectives: A Newsletter for Individuals with Alzheimer's Disease (phone: 858-622-5800).

Index